WHEN SOMEONE IN YOUR FAMILY HAS CANCER

Toni L. Rocha

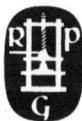

The Rosen Publishing Group, Inc.
New York

Published in 2001 by The Rosen Publishing Group, Inc.
29 East 21st Street, New York, NY 10010

First Edition

Cover photo © Stone

Library of Congress Cataloging-in-Publication Data

Rocha, Toni L.
   Coping when someone in your family has cancer / by Toni L. Rocha. — 1st ed.
       p.   cm.
Includes bibliographical references and index.
   ISBN: 978-1-4358-8646-9
   1. Cancer—Juvenile literature. 2. Adjustment (Psychology)—Juvenile literature. 3. Cancer—Psychological aspects—Juvenile literature. 4. Tumors in children—Juvenile literature. 5. Cancer—Patients—Family relationships—Juvenile literature. [1. Cancer—Psychological aspects. 2. Diseases—Psychological aspects.] I. Title.
   RC264 .R63 2000
   616.99'4—dc21
                                                    00-010319

Manufactured in the United States of America

About the Author

Toni L. Rocha retired in December 1999 from her position as police and fire reporter for the *Beloit Daily News* in Beloit, Wisconsin. With more than thirty years experience writing in various areas of the communications field, including advertising, she is now writing freelance from her home in Roscoe, Illinois. When she is not camped out in front of the computer, Toni travels, works counted cross-stitch, takes nature photographs, renders pen-and-ink drawings, carves wood, creates miniatures, gardens, and reads a lot.

Acknowledgments

This book is dedicated to Alex Salisbury and Matthew White, who have faced the worst a cancer diagnosis can bring with courage and fortitude. It is also dedicated to their families, most particularly Ellen Salisbury and Sheri White—two mothers who have also faced the worst life can bring and who have risen far above it.

Contents

Contents

Introduction

"It's simply not fair" is often our first reaction to news that someone we love has been diagnosed with cancer. Powerful and overwhelming emotions such as shock, guilt, anger, fear, and helplessness—a combination of all, or a pairing of a few—may be among the first feelings you'll experience. And often there's little comfort to be found in the realization that you're not alone.

The national statistics are grim. One of every two men, and one of every three women, will have cancer in his or her lifetime. Nearly 1.4 million Americans will be diagnosed with cancer this year alone. According to the National Coalition for Cancer, 538,000 people will die this year from cancer. That's one person every fifty-eight seconds. More than 10,000 of those diagnosed with cancer in the next year will be children. And you're right. It's not fair.

What may seem worse to you is that the majority of these people could have avoided being diagnosed with cancer. Almost 75 percent of all cancer cases in the United States are related to tobacco and alcohol abuse, and diet, according to the American Cancer Society. Less than 10 percent of all cancers can be related to environmental factors.

However, there are some encouraging signs in the struggle to cure cancer. Only thirty years ago, 33 percent of those diagnosed with cancer survived. Today, patients have a better than even chance as the survival rate edges toward 60 percent. Also, whereas only 5 percent of children survived leukemia thirty years ago, today the survival rate is more than 70 percent. The same is true of many other cancers. The survival rate has improved from less than 10 percent to nearly 100 percent when some kinds of cancer are diagnosed early.

According to the American Cancer Society, there are more than 8.2 million people living today who have had cancer. The bad news remains that even when the person lives through the cancer, the process takes a terrible toll on both the patient and those who care about him or her. So many things change when someone has cancer. Life is seldom the same for the other members of the person's family, regardless of the outcome.

In an odd way, cancer is similar to childhood diseases such as measles, chicken pox, and mumps. You may remember that when one child in your home caught a contagious disease, you and your other siblings probably caught it, too. You can't catch cancer, of course. But coping with cancer in your family may almost feel as if you had "caught" it.

This book has been written to help you cope with the challenges and feelings that naturally occur when someone you love is diagnosed with cancer. You'll read about people your age who are coping with cancer in their families, whether it's a brother, sister, parent, grandparent, or other relative. You'll also hear from medical professionals, support group leaders, social service volunteers, and adult family members who will share their insight and experience with cancer, as well as the effect that it has on family and friends. Getting through such difficult times as holidays, and how to say good-bye—should it become inevitable—are also subjects addressed in upcoming chapters.

You'll find many resources to supplement your quest for more information and support. But mostly this book is designed to guide you through difficult times and to help you face the painful, day-to-day reality of cancer recovery.

Overcoming Those First Fears

Just hearing the word "cancer" touches all of our emotions. As you can imagine, or may already know firsthand, a diagnosis of cancer in someone we know and love can be devastating. All the fears, worries, and even grief begin when we first hear the news.

In this book, you will read about Alex and Matt, two young patients who were diagnosed with cancer. Their mothers will share with you what happened during the period of time just before and after their sons were diagnosed.

How Alex's Story Began

Alex loved sports. The seventeen-year-old high school senior had played baseball since he was five years old. With his senior year about to begin, Alex's parents agreed to let him play varsity football. Alex's mother, Ellen, said that prior to his being a senior, she and Alex's father hadn't wanted him to play football because they worried that their son would be injured in some way that would prevent him from achieving his dream of playing baseball in college.

In late summer 1997, Alex began football practice. Despite the intense heat and humidity that August, Alex thrived on the experience. He enjoyed being part of a team, and he worked hard. During one of his practices, he took a hard hit to the ribs. Alex didn't think much of it, but the hit left him very sore. Within a few days, he began coughing up blood.

Alone, Alex went to the doctor's office to have his ribs and lungs checked. Part of that examination included taking a blood sample. A couple of days later, the doctor's office called and asked him to come in for a second blood test.

"They told Alex the results were unusual, possibly a laboratory error, and they wanted to double-check it themselves," Ellen said.

Meanwhile, Alex didn't get to play the season's first football game that Friday night. He stood on the side-lines, cheering for his team.

The next day, Alex went back to the doctor's office for still more blood tests.

"To the rest of us, he seemed fine," Ellen said. "His chest was still sore, but considering the hit, we thought that was normal."

When Alex's doctor called Sunday afternoon, Ellen said she knew the news wouldn't be good. Alex's uncle had died at age ten from acute lymphocytic leukemia, a cancer common to children.

"When he explained the results of the blood tests, I immediately asked if it was leukemia," Ellen added. "He told me it could be, but without a bone marrow biopsy, we wouldn't know for sure."

The one thing the doctor stressed was that Alex was in danger of infection and had to be hospitalized immediately. There, the doctors performed a bone marrow biopsy.

You probably have had blood tests. But not many people know what a bone marrow biopsy is like. A long, stainless steel syringe is inserted into the pelvic bone from either the front or the back. Marrow, which looks like blood but is thicker, is taken out of the bone, along with bone chips. Then tests are run on all the samples. This is what the doctors did with Alex.

> *"Alex received his diagnosis around noon on September 1, 1997," Ellen said. "I was the only other person with him. Dr. Nora at Rockford Memorial Hospital came into the room and told us Alex had acute non-lymphocytic leukemia, a cancer that's normally found in men age fifty and older. He said it wasn't the best diagnosis, but it wasn't the worst either."*
>
> *After apologizing for giving them such bad news, the doctor left them alone in the hospital room.*
>
> *"Alex cried for a few moments. I don't even think his tears lasted five minutes," Ellen said. "Then he pulled himself together and said he'd deal with it— he'd get through it. He never said 'why me?' Not that day."*
>
> *Ellen went home alone, to break the news to the rest of the family—Alex's father and three younger brothers. They cried, too.*

How Matt's Story Began

Matt hadn't been feeling well for a while. The lively two-year-old just wasn't himself. His mother, Sheri, and father, Greg, took him for a series of tests to find out just what was troubling their toddler.

"We went in on a Monday for an MRI (magnetic resonance imaging) to rule out a brain stem tumor," Sheri said. *"They had prepared us for the procedure by indicating that Matt would be put to sleep for the MRI. Then we would go to the pediatric floor to wait while Matt recovered from the anesthesia. After Matt woke up, we would be discharged, and the doctor would call us with the results. The fact of the matter is, it didn't quite go like that,"* Sheri said.

Following the MRI, before Matt was back with his parents, the nurse practitioner said the neurologist would go over the results with them.

"This didn't faze my husband and me," Sheri explained. *"It didn't even occur to us that there was a problem, even though they had first told us he would call with the results."*

When the doctor told Sheri and Greg something like, "I am sorry, your son's MRI indicates he has a brain tumor. He will be admitted to the pediatric ward, and he will need to have surgery. I will contact the surgeon now and he will come up and talk to you," Sheri said they began to realize that Matt was in serious trouble.

"We couldn't believe this. In fact, I'm not sure we even absorbed all he said," Sheri recalled. *"I remember my husband went back to look at the scans. The technicians and neurologist showed him the tumor on the scans. It took me until the next day or so to realize that when they said 'malignant brain tumor' it meant cancer."*

Sheri and Greg made a lot of phone calls those next few hours.

"Through our tears, we assured everyone we didn't need anyone to come up to the hospital with us," Sheri added. "But two of our best friends came up anyway, and really, we actually needed that."

Sheri and Greg cried for a long time. Sheri said her tears weren't really for the thought of cancer, as much as they were for the uncertainty and fear of not knowing what to expect. Seeing how critically ill Matt was following the surgery reinforced Sheri's fears.

"The pediatric oncologist, a specialist in child cancer, met with us that same afternoon and briefly described what his role would be in the next few years!" Sheri exclaimed. "He explained the 'Make-A-Wish' program. I declared I didn't want to do that. I would take my kid to Disney World when I wanted to and not because he was dying."

The doctor told Sheri and Greg that the Wish programs were not just for terminally ill children, and that corporations had put a lot of money into such programs, and all kids with life-threatening illnesses were entitled.

"There was that term—'life-threatening,'" Sheri said. "It was beginning to sink in that our son's surgery, scheduled for the next morning, was not your routine tonsillectomy."

However, it still seemed to Sheri and Greg that this was just a bump in the road.

"We would take care of this obstacle and move on," Sheri added. "I remember calling our church and asking them to tell our priest that the little two-year-old boy with red hair at 8:30 mass would be having brain tumor surgery in the morning and to please pray."

Because Matt's surgery left him so completely changed, cancer seemed secondary to the problem of seeing their son unable to do the things he could do prior to the surgery. Before the surgery, Matt had been sitting up, taking his pacifier in and out of his mouth, talking or crying, just as a normal toddler could.

"We did not know this child as ours anymore," Sheri said. *"But my husband said he was in there somewhere, and slowly but surely Matt would be making his way back to us."*

Getting Through the Diagnosis Stage

After seeing a doctor for the first time, there may be days or even weeks of uncertainty for a cancer patient and his or her family. There may be many more tests and possible hospitalization, just as in Alex's story. Or the doctors may find the cancer through advanced diagnostic methods such as an MRI. If the cancer is operable, an operation will probably be scheduled right away, depending on the patient's overall health. Alex's and Matt's stories are typical of how a patient learns he or she has cancer. The person develops a suspicious symptom, as Alex and Matt did, or finds one of cancer's warning signs.

The diagnosis stage is a tough time for everyone— patient, family, and friends. All kinds of thoughts and worries will go through your head, just as they will for the person awaiting diagnosis. Even after you hear the diagnosis, you'll be faced with even more questions and concerns, just as Alex's and Matt's families were.

"Alex was lucky," Ellen said. "He hadn't demonstrated any symptoms of his leukemia. If not for the blood test, we wouldn't have known until symptoms started to occur."

Ellen said their first worry was whether or not Alex's cancer had been caught early enough. The oncologist, a cancer specialist, who diagnosed Alex told his family he thought Alex was between three and six months of the leukemia's onset. Did catching it early make a difference?

"For Alex, it made a difference because he was stronger," Ellen said. "After his workouts in the weight room, getting into condition for football, Alex weighed 210 pounds. At six feet, five inches, that was just right."

Waiting for and Receiving the Diagnosis

Sometimes the patient who is waiting for a diagnosis may want to confide in you. It eases the patient's anxiety, but it won't be easy for you. You'll have to put aside all your fears and worries while you're talking with the patient. Do your best to remain upbeat, positive, and calm. The most helpful thing you can do is to listen without questioning, guessing, or jumping to any conclusions.

Most of all, it's important to help the patient keep his or her hopes up. Waiting for test results, plus that painful time when the person first hears the diagnosis, is hard on everyone involved. Being there for the person, even when you can't do anything except hold hands and listen with a shared sense of optimism, can help ease the burden.

As in Alex's case, the doctor is the person who provides the patient with a diagnosis. You may learn about the cancer diagnosis before the patient, either because someone tells you or because you overhear the sad news. This can easily happen if the patient is a very young child—a kid brother or sister to you or a friend. Either way, difficult as it might be, keep it to yourself.

It is up to the doctor to determine if the patient should be told right away. He or she also decides when the patient should be told the news and how much information about the illness the patient can handle at that time. The overall welfare of the patient comes first.

"Most often, when a patient comes in for a diagnosis, he or she has a strong feeling about what may be wrong," explained Karen Gessner, a licensed cancer social worker in the Center for Cancer at OSF Saint Anthony Medical Center, in Rockford, Illinois. "If it's an adult, he or she almost always brings a family member for support. Rarely are teenagers included in the diagnosis meeting."

"That might be a disservice," Karen added, "because then children don't hear the news firsthand. And when parents or grandparents come home from the hospital, they may feel too overwhelmed to be able to talk about what is going on with their children."

"Even very young children know when something is wrong," Karen said. "And it's natural for adults to want to protect the younger family members. But they do need to know. Otherwise, their imaginations may run rampant and they'll start to believe it's worse than it really may be. I believe honesty is the best policy."

The manner in which the news is given can differ widely from case to case. When the doctor talks with the patient and a member of the family at the same time, it gives the patient a feeling of confidence that the truth is being told and that no one is withholding information.

Some adult cancer patients may prefer to be told privately, while others need to have a shared discussion. It's up to the patient to decide, and that decision should be respected.

Although your first impulse might be to protect your family member from distressing news, it's best to be honest. This is true especially if the patient is a very young brother or sister. Problems that result from not being honest and open with the patient from the start could make the situation worse. This could cause the patient to feel isolated and more afraid of what he or she is not being told.

On the other hand, you need to take care that you don't go too far when you talk with the patient. In any case, it's important to be sure that whatever you say to the patient is truthful. Otherwise, the patient will eventually lose trust in the people he or she needs most.

Karen also pointed out that it's important not to just announce bad news. "One thing that helps is hearing there's a plan in place to help the patient recover," Karen said. "It is also helpful to stress that the child, regardless of age, is not responsible in any way for the illness. The child might feel guilty and wonder what he or she did to cause this. The answer is 'nothing.'"

How much the doctor tells the patient at the beginning of the diagnosis, and how much information is added at each point in the treatment plan, depends on what the doctor thinks the patient is ready to handle—obviously, a lot depends on the age of the cancer victim. Doctors also take the family's feelings into consideration.

When dealing with doctors, it's not unusual to feel that you have questions that aren't being answered to your satisfaction. Karen advises that you never hesitate to ask, but be cautious about asking the patient questions. He or she may not be ready to answer tough questions. Your parents might not be either. That's when you may want to turn to other family members, a teacher or school counselor, or maybe even a friend who has a family member being treated for cancer.

Sources of Support

"Cancer support meetings are another good way to learn more about cancer and its treatment," Karen added. "But because many of these meetings include adults, sometimes it takes teens longer to open up. You can always talk to hospital social workers, the chaplain, and nurses. The doctor might wait to see how much you want to know before he or she gives you answers."

Another source of good information is your local chapter of the American Cancer Society. The society has dozens of books available that offer information on a level that is appropriate for teens and children. The public library is another place where you can find books and pamphlets on coping when someone in your family is diagnosed with cancer. You'll find many resources in the Where to Go for Help section in the back of this book.

"I'd caution teens about searching for information about cancer on the Internet," Karen added. "Some of what they might find is terrifying."

In upcoming chapters, you'll continue to read about how Alex's and Matt's families coped with their cancers.

When Cancer
Strikes a Parent

When we are younger, we often look up to our parents and older family members (older siblings, close cousins, and aunts or uncles) as invulnerable leaders and role models. It's a painful shock when someone in our family is diagnosed with cancer. Like having a rug pulled from beneath your feet, the impact of such unwelcome news can leave you stunned and disoriented.

Having cancer can be a terrible and lonely experience. No one, regardless of age, should have to bear it alone. Parents and grandparents who try to keep their cancer diagnoses a secret rob their loved ones of the opportunity to express love, concern, and support. By sharing the diagnosis, the patient and his or her family and friends can begin to create a strong foundation of mutual understanding and trust.

After your parent or other close family member is diagnosed with cancer, doctors and social workers believe that giving you the correct information about the diagnosis and how the cancer will be treated is the most important step in guiding you toward coming to terms with this situation.

Why Pretending Nothing Is Wrong Is a Bad Idea

"No matter what the child's age, a parent's best bet is to be honest," advised Patty Kirkham, an oncology social worker for Rockford Health Services in Rockford, Illinois. "Trying to hide what's happening is the worst mistake parents can make."

Parents often believe that they can shield their children from knowing about a diagnosis as long as they are able to act as though nothing out of the ordinary has happened. This isn't possible, of course. Life is far from normal for a family coping with a cancer diagnosis. It can be very stressful for a parent to keep a cancer diagnosis secret.

Also, we can usually tell if our parents are worried without having to be told. Even very young children sense when something is wrong. However, when your whole world is turned upside down and whispered conversations go on behind closed doors, it's easy at any age to believe you're the cause of all the trouble, or to imagine much worse situations.

"Like most teens, you are probably somewhat aware of cancer," Patty added. "You hear about cancer, its treatments, and statistics on television. You can read about it in newspapers, or in books, or you can easily find dozens of Web sites about cancer and its treatment on the Internet."

"The best thing teens can do if they believe their parents are shielding them from a painful truth is to ask questions," Patty said. "Tell your parents you want to be involved in every part of their treatment. What you know is easier to face than the unknown. If they still hesitate to open their hearts and discuss their fears, insist on being included."

They may not be ready to believe it at first, but your parents just might feel more in control of themselves and their lives when they are able to deal openly with your questions and concerns. Because a parent's priority is to help his or her children cope with life, you and your parents may actually feel relief when you begin to tackle the issue together. Honest communication between you and your sick parent is vital throughout the course of the illness.

"It might help to develop a slogan you and your parents can use to help focus on coping together, such as 'As a family, we can cope with this,'" Patty added. "The alternative to honesty and coping can be serious trouble. There are two ways teens tend to behave after a parent is diagnosed with cancer," Patty explained. "One is to ask questions and participate in the recovery process. The other is to isolate themselves. That's when trouble can start."

You should be aware that it will be hard to watch as your cancer-stricken relative gains or loses weight, loses his or her hair, or is unable to eat. Oncology social workers believe it's important for you to understand how your parent's cancer is going to be treated and what side effects your parent is likely to have.

You'll read about cancer treatments and what can happen to patients afterward in chapter 4. Many hospitals and cancer treatment centers offer group support meetings for children, teens, and adults. Attending these meetings is a good way to meet other teens who are going through the same family crisis you are. Together, you can share experiences, learn how other teens are coping with cancer in their families, and support one another.

As Patty said, "Sharing what's happening with your mother or father takes away a lot of the strangeness and helps you to be comfortable."

Dealing with Your Feelings

Another challenge you might face is the angry feelings of the parent or relative who is ill. This anger can be a reaction to feeling sick—a different "why me?" response. Sadly, it's often those who are the closest to the ill person who are the targets of this frustration and anger. Whether or not this anger is directed at you or at another family member, it's important to try not to take it personally.

If it all becomes too much to bear alone, turn to people who can help you deal with your feelings. Talking to an understanding friend can help, even if it's just to vent your own frustration and fears. Talking about your troubles—with a teacher you trust, a school counselor, a religious mentor, or an oncology social worker at the hospital or clinic where your parent is being treated—is a positive way to ease the anguish you may be feeling.

Teens who feel isolated from what is happening within their families might begin to hang around with the wrong crowd or get into trouble at school or in other ways. This sort of behavior is a cry for attention that needs to be addressed immediately.

A parent who suddenly becomes childlike and dependent is demonstrating another common reaction to receiving a diagnosis of cancer. This sort of regressive behavior is a way of letting the rest of the family know that the victim doesn't feel up to coping with the illness.

You may find yourself feeling extremely protective of your parent. Hard as it may sound, this is not a useful reaction. At this point, it's good to remember that any person fighting cancer, regardless of age, is better off if he or she is able to remain involved in the normal rhythms of family life. What your parent really needs is understanding and help, not sympathy or overindulgence.

You may need to take on more responsibilities at home than you have in the past. It will help you get through some of the more difficult times if you understand that this is a temporary situation. Your parents are relying on your extra help until they can resume their roles. You may have to miss a basketball game or school dance, a movie or an outing with your friends. However, it's equally important to avoid spending all your time thinking about, and worrying about, your parent's illness.

Attending school every day, no matter how fearful you might feel about leaving home, helps because it gives you time away from home and something else to think about besides your parent's cancer. Also, at school, you will be with friends whose support and understanding is much more beneficial than being isolated at home.

Don't be surprised or shocked if your healthy parent asks you for extra help for a short period of time so that he or she may have some time off from being the primary caregiver. A mother or father who has become a caregiver needs occasional breaks to help maintain emotional and physical well-being. Your parent may ask another family member, a close friend, or a visiting nurse to help for an afternoon or a day so that he or she can get out of the house or rest without being disturbed. What being away at school during the day does for you, having an afternoon off can do for your healthy parent.

One of the hardest things about coping with cancer in your family is maintaining your balance and perspective.

It's too easy to get deeply mired in thoughts of treatments, side effects, hospitalization, and sickness. If you find yourself slipping into this state of mind, a good way to lift your spirits is to ask a close friend to visit or, if you can leave the house for an hour or two, go to that friend's home.

Once the two of you are together, make a pact not to talk about your parent's illness. Instead, spend the time talking about normal subjects, play a computer game, or do homework together. Just one hour spent doing the things you've always done with your friend can raise your spirits. Laugh a lot, tell jokes, be yourself.

More than ever before, you might find yourself responsible for how much sleep you get, how well you eat, and other aspects of your life that you may have depended on your parents to regulate. Coping with cancer in the family can be a maturing experience, no matter what your age. Never hesitate to ask for help when you begin to feel overwhelmed. That's what family and friends are for.

Much of what you just have read about coping with a parent's cancer applies to coping with a brother or sister who has cancer. You'll learn more about that kind of coping when you read chapter 3.

When Cancer
Strikes a Brother or
Sister

In chapter 1, you read about Alex, a high school senior who was diagnosed with leukemia just as school began. Here is more of his story as told by his mother, Ellen.

Coming to Terms with Alex's Cancer

"Between September and December that year, a lot happened," Ellen said. *"Alex's three younger brothers—Forrest, Daniel, and Lucas—had to come to terms with their brother's potentially terminal illness. They visited Alex in the hospital but only as often as Alex would allow. If he was feeling really sick, he didn't want any visitors. I was the only person he wanted with him.*

"Alex's brothers cried when they first heard the news, and then they went about doing what they needed to do, had to do, and wanted to do.

"Alex was always there in their minds, along with his illness. Decisions were sometimes made around Alex. It was important for them to spend time with him. No one knew what was going to happen or how long Alex would have."

Forrest, the next oldest in the family, became the source of information on Alex's condition at high school. It was okay in the beginning, but Forrest had a very hard time focusing on tedious things like schoolwork, unless it was a real hands-on project. He has had to change his courses almost every semester since Alex's diagnosis.

"Forrest played a lot more video/strategy games and stuck closer to home. He opted out of parties and other social events so he'd have more time with Alex. Forrest quit football in his senior year because of the time required for practice and the coach's lack of sensitivity to what was going on at home.

"Forrest wasn't sleeping well. Migraines became a big problem, causing Forrest to miss school.

"Meanwhile, the next youngest brother, Danny, kept his worries to himself and didn't want to talk about Alex's illness at all. Instead, he spent a lot of time with Alex when he was home between chemotherapy treatments and infections that required hospitalization. Together, Alex and Danny played video games and watched sports on television.

"Ironically, Danny 'grew up,' going from a temper-tantrum teen to a maturing young man who helped me more without the usual griping. He didn't like or want to talk about Alex's diagnosis. There were times when he'd stay away from home as much as possible after school and during weekends. But at other times," Ellen continued, "Danny wanted to be around all the time. When Alex returned from out-of-state treatment and spent three weeks in the hospital, Danny spent a lot of overnights in Alex's room.

"During that time, Alex had little or no control over his bladder and bowels. Danny helped change Alex, and he made no insulting or degrading comments. Danny spent almost the whole summer after Alex's diagnosis with his grandmother, not returning until August. Alex had been in remission from his leukemia when Danny left, but relapsed in late July. Danny was extremely irritated that he hadn't been told about his older brother's declining condition and that he hadn't been around to help.

"Danny coped pretty well with the situation. He maintained his grades without any major lapses. He had also been more of a loner than the others, and stayed that way through Alex's illness. He also had trouble sleeping at night. The youngest, Lucas, probably had the hardest time of all because of his age and the relationship—or lack thereof—he had with Alex," Ellen recalled. "Lucas at first acted as if he planned to ignore the entire situation. He didn't want to know or see anything.But after a month or so, Lucas became the most inquisitive and wanted to learn how to help Alex, including flushing his lines and changing his site dressing. He asked a lot of questions about Alex's care, treatment, and prognosis.

"Although Alex appreciated Lucas's offer, he wasn't comfortable with Lucas taking care of that for him. Nor did Lucas spend much time with Alex when he was hospitalized. Alex had less tolerance for Lucas because of his age and maturity level. That bothered Lucas because he wanted to be closer. A family friend recently told us that Lucas had a crying episode in school, something Lucas never told us.

"Lucas continued to try to find ways to spend time with Alex at home. He ended up spending his time at home trying to deal with why Alex was rejecting his help

"Both my husband and I tried talking to Alex about this point a number of times but couldn't make any headway. We're not sure whether Alex understood. We also tried to explain to Lucas the nature of what was taking place within Alex, that it was the illness that was affecting his brain. But we knew that no amount of explaining would remedy the hurt.

"Still, during the time Alex spent at home, Lucas would offer to wheel Alex or bring him things Alex couldn't get himself, such as drinks, snacks, or even medications. Lucas never made degrading remarks or showed any shame over the fact that his brother couldn't use a toilet like everyone else in the family.

"Holidays and special events became milestones for Alex and our family. Each one reached was a victory over the leukemia. One of Alex's major goals was attending his senior prom.

"Originally, Alex planned to go to the prom by himself. One of his best friends, Tracy, wasn't planning to go either. Her boyfriend had graduated the year before. However, after some discussion, the two decided to go together.

"Forrest acted as chaperone and 'bouncer' for the event. Alex and Forrest were the highlight of the prom when they danced to the Village People's recording of 'YMCA' with Alex riding on Forrest's shoulders. Forrest wasn't intimidated by carrying his brother, nor was Alex intimidated by being carried. That part of their relationship was to become very important."

Matt's Family: Tired of All the Crying

You read about Matt, the toddler recovering from a brain tumor, in chapter 1. His mother, Sheri, said that his older brother, Joey, just four years old when Matt was diagnosed, was too young to really become involved directly. However, he did strongly express his disapproval at how his home life was being disrupted.

"One night, Joey came into the darkened kitchen where I was talking about Matt to a good high school friend," Sheri said. "He said 'Mommy, I'm tired of all the crying. When are you going to stop?'"

The tears have lessened since that night, Sheri said, but they haven't stopped.

What You Can Do

The impact of a cancer diagnosis is staggering when the patient is your brother or sister. You will probably feel shock, anger, numbness, and even guilt. You'll wonder why it has to be *your* brother or sister, and why now.

Suddenly, life is filled with hospital visits and conversations about clinics, tests and treatments, strange medical jargon, and uncertainty. Your home life will no doubt be disrupted. And because of the treatments, your previously healthy sibling may now be bald, tired, and frequently very sick. He or she may be in the hospital for days or for weeks. Sadness and worry are two emotions that you'll experience during these difficult times.

As you have just read, Alex's and Matt's siblings each reacted differently to the reality of needing to cope with their brothers' cancers. Unlike their parents, your parents might not want to talk about a sibling's sickness or answer your questions. That's not surprising, according to Patty Kirkham, the oncology social worker at Rockford Health Services.

After the Diagnosis—When Emotions Run High

"After a child is diagnosed with cancer, parents are often a complete wreck. If you feel that you need more information than your parents have given you, it's okay to ask your brother or sister what he or she knows," Patty said. "Your brother or sister might need to share what he or she knows about the illness, along with his or her fears. And if, after you've talked together, you both feel you need clarification on any point, the two of you can go to your parents and ask them to sit down and talk about the situation openly and honestly."

There are negative feelings besides fear, grief, and worry that you may have to confront as well. You might feel guilty. You may wonder if you did or said something to your brother or sister that caused this terrible disease in your brother or sister. It might surprise you to learn that parents often feel this way, too.

But just because you think or wish something, it doesn't necessarily happen. People often wish bad things would happen when they're angry at another person. The important thing to remember is that no one really knows for certain exactly why children, or even adults, get cancer. But one thing is certain—nothing you said or did caused it.

"Another difficult issue that festers in teens is anger," Patty said. "Teens tend to believe they are at the center of their world, and they resent it when they're not able to continue their lives as usual. First they get angry after a family member is diagnosed with cancer, and then they feel guilty about it. It's okay to be angry. That realization is a great relief for teens coping with cancer in their families.

"You're human," Patty stressed. "It will take a great deal of weight off your mind to know that everyone feels that way at some point. It's part of the grieving process, and it's perfectly natural. What's important is that you recognize and accept the way you feel. The next important thing is how you deal with those feelings.

"A lot depends on family," Patty added. "The worst possible case would be for a teen to punish himself or herself for those seemingly uncontrollable negative feelings. It's important to confront your anger and guilt. Finding someone to talk to about your feelings is a good way to start. Social workers, parents, school counselors, good friends, and the pastor at your church can help."

Jealousy is another emotion that you may feel. After all, a sibling who can miss school, or get a lot of extra attention, especially from Mom and Dad, may seem lucky. To top it off, sick kids often get lots of presents, even when it's not their birthday or a holiday. However, it's important to realize that no matter how it seems, your sick sibling is not enjoying being sick.

Even though this type of jealousy is often quite petty, it does frequently occur. Siblings of a sick patient can feel jealous. They also can feel that they're being left out, or think that their parents love the sick child more. And these kinds of very complicated feelings are difficult to overcome, especially since they are probably not logical.

If you feel jealous, the best thing you can do is find someone you trust and talk it out. Bringing these kinds of emotions out into the open and dealing with them as they surface will do you the greatest good in the long run. It is also important to realize that even if the jealousy seems unreasonable, it is a natural reaction. Making someone feel guilty about their jealous feelings will only make matters worse.

Worry may be another emotion you may encounter. It hurts to see your sibling lose his or her hair, gain or lose weight, and not feel like playing or sometimes even talking. You might feel guilty about feeling good, about being able to go out and do things like in-line skating, bikeriding, and swimming while your brother or sister is stuck at home or in the hospital.

When Your Parents Seem Less Available
Another thing that will be difficult to deal with is the fact that you may not have as much access to your parents as before. "Your parents might be preoccupied, but it's okay to remind them that you're here and need attention, too. Getting more involved in the treatment and recovery process can lift you above those feelings and give you something positive to do," Patty said.

Usually, when a child is in the hospital, one or both of the parents stay with him or her or spend a lot of time with him or her. You may have to stay with family or friends during these times, especially if the hospital or treatment clinic isn't close to home. If you have other siblings, they may have to stay in other homes. Being cut off from the patient and from your parents can be frightening, frustrating, and can cause a lot of anguish.

You can alleviate these feelings of isolation by scheduling daily telephone calls when you all know where you'll be. If you are too far away and the calls are long-distance, keep in touch by e-mail at home, at a relative's home, or through your school or local library. Just knowing that you can talk to each other every day will help ease the anxiety of feeling apart from what is happening in your family.

However, don't worry. Things usually do settle down after a few weeks. Children usually don't stay in the hospital longer than that, and follow-up treatment is usually by appointment at clinics or the doctor's office. Sometimes, chemotherapy or radiation treatments are performed at the hospital, but the sibling won't be there for very long.

The Importance of Trying to Maintain a Normal Routine

It is important for families to try to continue their normal routine. This not only helps you, but it helps the patient, too. Because the illness affects everyone around him or her, your sick sibling may feel guilty about keeping you from doing the things you love. Once your sibling recovers or goes into remission from the cancer, he or she will then be able to participate in more activities.

School may seem unimportant, for you as well as for the patient, but it offers a place to grow, both socially and intellectually. School is also the place where you can look to the future with optimism.

In major cancer centers, 50 to 75 percent of children are being saved, from acute leukemia, 90 percent from Wilms' tumor (a cancer or the kidneys), 75 percent from Hodgkin's disease, and 70 to 80 percent, from bone cancer.

Most pediatric oncologists—specialists who treat children's cancers—recommend that children participate in regular school activities as soon as possible after treatment. At first, this may be scary. You may feel the need to protect your sick sibling. You may be concerned that the other children will make fun of the changes treatment has caused. You may even fear your friends will crack unkind jokes about your sick sibling.

But going to school reinforces your sibling's need to belong. Pediatric oncologists strongly believe that children need school because it's where their friends are. And school offers a natural way to bring your brother's or sister's life back to normal.

Being the brother or sister of someone with cancer can seem really hard. After all, cancer is a serious, complex disease and the treatments necessary to deal with it may seem harsh to the point of almost not being worth the pain and misery they cause. To make matters worse, you may feel that there is nothing that you can do to help your ill sibling. However, this is not at all true.

Do not forget that there are millions of seemingly little things you can do that will make your sibling feel cared for. For example, one teen began making "welcome home" cards for his little sister each time she returned from the hospital. He left the colorful cards with funny or loving messages on his sister's pillow in her room where she would find them immediately. It gave her something special to come home to, while her brother felt that he was helping her get well by keeping her spirits up.

Remember, through all the pain and uncertainty, that your parents love you, too, and want to help with any problems you may be having dealing with a brother or sister who has cancer. Let them know how you feel so that you can deal with those feelings more effectively.

Understanding Chemotherapy and Other Treatments

Learning that a family member has cancer is a difficult thing to deal with. Witnessing the effects that chemotherapy and other treatments may have on your family member may be harder still. When you know what to expect and how chemotherapy helps despite outward appearances, you will be better able to put aside your fears and concentrate on supporting the patient.

The number of treatment options depends on what type of cancer your family member has. Age, physical condition, and personal preferences are also factors in the decision to use one treatment over another.

The Four Main Treatment Types

According to information provided by the American Cancer Society, there are generally four major types of cancer treatments: surgery, radiation, chemotherapy, and biological therapies. Bone marrow transplants and hormone therapy are two other possibilities.

A. Surgery has traditionally been the first treatment choice for many kinds of cancer. About 60 percent of cancer patients have surgery. When the cancer is localized—found in just one place, as in Matt's brain stem tumor—surgery is used to remove it, along with surrounding tissue which might contain cancer cells. About 30 percent of patients are cured with surgery alone. For the rest, a regime of either radiation or chemotherapy is added before and/or after the surgery to ensure the cancer is gone.

B. Radiation is used for localized cancers, too. Radiation therapy can destroy or damage cancer cells so that the cells are unable to multiply. More than 50 percent of cancer patients have radiation treatment at some point. This treatment is delivered either through external high-energy rays or through internal implants. External radiation is painless and is done on an out-patient basis. Implants, small containers of radiation placed in or near the tumor, allow the patient to receive a higher total dose of radiation in a smaller area. Some implants can be placed in an out-patient center while others may require hospitalization for a few days.

The most common side effects from radiation therapy can include fatigue, skin changes in the area being treated, and some loss of appetite. If the radiation treatment is done on the patient's head, he or she might become temporarily bald. These side effects will eventually go away.

C. Chemotherapy is used to treat cancer that has spread throughout the patient's body, or for cancers such as leukemia. Depending on the type of cancer and its development stage, chemotherapy can be used to cure cancer, to prevent it from spreading, to slow the cancer's growth, to kill cancer cells that may have spread to other parts of the patient's body, or to relieve symptoms caused by cancer.

Chemotherapy involves the use of powerful anticancer drugs injected directly into the patient's bloodstream or given by mouth. Nearly 100 different drugs can be used, individually or in combination. How many are used, as well as how they are combined, is what the oncologist must determine based on the patient's type of cancer, overall health, and prognosis.

Chemo treatments are given in cycles, followed by a recovery period, for about six months on average. Used after surgery, chemotherapy can significantly reduce the chance that the cancer will reoccur in another part of the patient's body or that it will return to the same site.

Side effects depend on the type and combination of drugs used, the amount taken, and the length of treatment. The most common and obvious is temporary hair loss, which can include not just the hair on the patient's head, but the eyebrows, eyelashes, mustache and beard, chest hair, underarm hair, and leg hair as well. Not every patient loses his or her hair, and it does grow back after chemo treatments stop.

Nausea and vomiting are another common side effect of chemotherapy. Don't be surprised if your family member refuses to eat, begins eating foods he or she normally doesn't like, or stops eating his or her favorite foods. This type of reaction varies widely, depending on the individual, but the patient will almost always go back to normal eating patterns after the chemotherapy is ended.

"Most kids experience feeding problems during chemo, most often because the gastrointestinal system is so wiped out from the drugs that food can't be tolerated," Matt's mother, Sheri, said. "Their taste buds are affected as well, so eating isn't as pleasurable."

Sheri added that mouth sores are also common, making it painful for some patients to eat at all. These eating problems are generally counteracted by the use of a nasal-gastric tube (n-g tube). This tube is inserted through the nose, down the throat, and into the stomach by a nurse or parent. Formula is generally what is fed through the n-g tube, which can be taken out each time or left in, especially during sessions of heavy chemotherapy.

"An n-g tube wasn't an option for us, as Matt's problems were more neurological than temporary side effects," Sheri explained.

A total nutrient solution called TPN may be fed to the patient by IV if he or she cannot eat normally. TPN looks like a large bag of milk, and contains all the nutrients and calories a patient needs. Sheri said TPN is often referred to as "steak and potatoes in a bag."

"Matt needed TPN for about six months during those first heavy chemotherapy treatments because he couldn't even tolerate the formula feeds," Sheri added. "TPN is usually a last resort to nourish the patient, as it can be damaging to some organs, such as the liver."

The physical changes caused by cancer and its treatments can be very hard to accept. Hair loss is one obvious side effect, but there are others that are just as radical. Your family member may lose weight, especially muscle, because he or she is not as active. Arms and legs may become thin and flabby. Some medications can make the patient's face or other body part swell. Some cancers, such as liver cancer, can cause the abdomen to swell significantly.

Alex's mother, Ellen, mentioned infertility as another possible side effect of chemotherapy. She mentioned that some pediatric oncologists and hematologists (blood specialists) are reluctant to discuss infertility with teens.

"Too many, including Alex, have learned the results too late. That can cause a major emotional upset," Ellen added. "Patients in the fifteen- to eighteen-year-old bracket need to know about this possibility in order to make informed decisions about their cancer treatment."

An increased chance of infection because of the patient's lower immunity, and fatigue are two more common side effects. You may have to limit the number of friends or relatives you can bring into the home to prevent the patient from catching a cold or the flu. Changes may need to be made in how your home is cleaned. Your ill family member may want to sleep a lot and have no energy for his or her favorite activities. These side effects are also temporary.

Some side effects are worse than others, and not every patient will experience each of these symptoms. But most can be controlled with medications, supportive care measures, or by changing the treatment schedule if necessary.

Hard as it is to see your loved one suffer through harsh chemical treatments, it's important to keep in mind that the long-term benefits should outweigh the misery. Some side effects can become chronic because the chemotherapy inhibits the patient's immune system and changes the chemical balance in his or her body. This can open the door to diseases unrelated to cancer. Diabetes is one possible result of taking steroid-based drugs such as prednisone, as an example.

D. Evidence suggests that the immune system plays a major role in the body's response to cancer. Biological therapies are promising new treatment methods for certain types of cancer. These treatments are somtimes classified as immunotherapy, biotherapy, or biological response modifiers. Simply put, biological therapies boost and support the body's immune system so it can fight cancer naturally, from within. This therapy can also lessen the side effects of more traditional cancer treatments.

Biological therapies can act in several ways: they can interfere with cancer cell growth; they can support healthy immune cells; in some cases, they provide cancer control; and they can help repair normal cells damaged by other forms of cancer treatment. There are several kinds of biological therapy in use now, being combined with radiation or chemotherapy treatments. You may have heard terms such as interleukins, interferons, or tumor necrosis factor used by the media to describe them.

When treatment is successful and the cancer is under control, the patient is in remission. In complete remission, all signs of the cancer disappear. Partial remission, in which the cancer shrinks but does not disappear, is also possible.

Remission can last from several weeks to many years. If the cancer comes back, another remission can often be induced with more treatment. Sometimes, it is necessary to use a different type of treatment the second time because the patient's cancer has developed resistance to the original therapy.

Alex's Experience with Chemotherapy and Bone Marrow Biopsies

As Told by His Mother, Ellen

"Alex never said 'why me?' the day he was diagnosed with leukemia. The only time he ever said it was after his first round of chemotherapy, when I brought him home from the hospital. He was so sick, he literally crawled up the stairs to his bed and cried, 'Why me?'

"I don't think anyone can ever be prepared for the effects of chemo, even a patient who has undergone it previously. Alex's first five days of chemo caused intense nausea and vomiting, and took away his appetite. His second five-day session after a brief break

in between caused less nausea. Alex was able to keep food down after the second session. Alex's theory on dealing with chemo and the effects was to sleep through it. The longer he slept, the faster time went by. He didn't feel he was missing anything because he was so miserable. In some ways, this was a blessing. And this was how Alex dealt with his last days.

"The purpose of chemotherapy is to kill off cancerous cells. Unfortunately, with blood-based cancers such as leukemia, by trying to kill off one kind of cell, the treatment kills off all the others. To stimulate a regrowth of white cells after chemo, a substance with the brand name Neupogen is injected directly under the skin. Throughout treatment, doctors conducted bone marrow biopsies to determine how the chemotherapy and injections were working.

"Alex's first bone marrow biopsy was done without any anesthesia, just a shot of Novocaine. When Alex learned that he could have had something more to help him get through it, he was ecstatic. This would be the one thing he'd want the world to know—that all patients needing bone marrow biopsies should be entitled to short-acting anesthesia. Typically, older children and adults are not even told of its use.

"Whenever he could, Alex had lumbar punctures, or spinal taps, done at the same time as the bone marrow biopsies in his hip. That way, he would be 'out' for them both. These two procedures allow doctors to draw fluids from the spinal column for testing. They require the patient to lie very still for long periods of time and can be very painful. Alex never suffered much pain from them afterward, but the scarring was very obvious—dimples about 1/16-inch deep were reminders of all the biopsies.

"For Alex's treatment, a central line was surgically implanted before his chemotherapy began. Placed in the chest just beneath the skin and connected to an artery, the central line is considered the best delivery method for chemotherapy." Alex's chemo was administered directly into the central line by an IV drip, which you may have seen used in TV shows about doctors and paramedics. Ellen said the reason the central line is connected to an artery in the chest rather than in an arm is that the arms' veins would disintegrate too quickly because of the strength of the drugs being used.

"Blood can be drawn out through the line as well as IV-delivered nutrients, medications, and blood transfusions introduced into the body, ending a multitude of painful needle sticks. It looked somewhat weird, this thin, white rubber line hanging out of Alex's chest with two valves on the end. What was even stranger was you could see the line rise over his clavicle in his chest, under the skin. Worst of all, Alex discovered it made a neat 'toy' to play with.

"Alex's central line had to be flushed out regularly with a saline solution and heparin, a chemical that keeps blood clots from forming. Because the line was exposed, it also had to have a dressing covering it, which needed to be changed every couple of days to prevent infection. This was the part of Alex's home care that his youngest brother, Lucas, offered to do.

"With his central line in place, Alex received his first chemotherapy session at the hospital. The chemo was fed into his bloodstream by an IV drip through *the implanted line. Then Alex was released to recover at home."* Even there, Ellen explained, Alex continued to receive chemo-based drugs four to six times each day through the central line.

"The line was left in his chest to facilitate future chemotherapy treatments, as well as the blood tests Alex needed regularly. Because Alex was nauseated and vomiting, normal saline solution was also IV-dripped into the central line to keep him hydrated." Ellen said a number of Alex's drugs couldn't be mixed —run through the central line at the same time. After each drug was given, Ellen flushed the line with saline solution before introducing the next dose.

"Alex kept his central line in place from his first chemotherapy treatment in the hospital in September 1997 until April 1998 when he had been in remission for about four months.

"A few days after he came home, Alex developed the first of many infections.

"Leukemia destroys the blood's white cells, the part that fights infection and makes the pus you see in infected wounds. Without sufficient white blood cells, Alex was extremely vulnerable to infections of all kinds. These infections can occur regardless of how carefully the patient is treated.

"With the infection came hospitalization. I think the first infection was the worst because we were all just learning what to expect from Alex's body and his strong will to beat the leukemia. As with most infections at this time in a patient's treatment, the type Alex had was never pinpointed. The good news was that antibiotics

worked on it, and the infection went away. Alex was released after five days. A couple of days later, Alex's white blood count went back up . . . the Neupogen had done its job.

"The normal range for white blood cell counts returning is between thirty and forty days. Alex's were back on day twenty-five. Very good news for everyone."

The Risk of Infection

As Alex continued with regularly scheduled rounds of chemotherapy, infections continued to occur. Sometimes Alex would also need blood transfusions to correct a low hemoglobin count. How he took care of his mouth and teeth became extremely important—brushing his teeth thoroughly and using a special mouth rinse called Peridex was vital.

"Between Alex's first and second rounds of chemo, he had a tooth extracted to prevent infection," his mother, Ellen, explained. "During his first round, he had developed a few sores, similar to canker sores, on the inside of his cheeks. Fortunately, those had healed without incident."

Ellen added that, to many of us, canker sores are something to tolerate even though they are painful. But for Alex, those sores took on a new meaning. At one point when his white blood cell count was very low, Alex developed what doctors call a "kissing sore." It started on the inside of Alex's cheek and "kissed" his gum opposite. The infection spread rapidly, and Alex was admitted to the hospital. Within a short period, his face was swollen to three times its normal size. He couldn't eat or talk. He couldn't tolerate the medical students and student nurses who had absolutely no clue what terrible pain he was dealing with.

Tests showed that the infection in Alex's mouth wasn't anything unusual. Only time would heal the sore that had spread until it encompassed the entire left side of Alex's face, including his lower jaw.

Alex's Remission and Relapse

"In January 1998, after five months of intensive chemotherapy treatments, Alex's leukemia went into remission. Alex's weight had dropped from 210 pounds at diagnosis to 155 pounds," Ellen said.

He still needed to see his oncologist every month for blood tests and remained on maintenance medications, but he was on his own. His central line, which had been in place since his first chemo treatment, was surgically removed in April. The family slowly began to get back to normal.

"But our summer was cut short on July 29, when a routine blood test revealed that Alex had relapsed— his leukemia was back.

"Alex cried. We all cried. Relapse had always lingered at the back of our minds, but the reality of it was overwhelming. Alex was admitted to the hospital. A new central line had to be placed, and a bone marrow biopsy done. Chemotherapy was scheduled to start immediately. But this time, the chemo protocol was different because it was based on the probability that Alex would need a bone marrow transplant.

According to the American Cancer Society, bone marrow transplants are done for three reasons:

1. In the case of bone marrow failure, the transplant replaces absent or abnormal cells with functional cells, allowing the natural production of blood cells to resume.

2. If the patient has cancer, as in Alex's case, the bone marrow transplant replaces cells that are killed as a side effect of high-dose chemotherapy and radiation therapy given to cure the cancer.

3. When genetic errors are present, the bone marrow transplant replaces defective or absent cells in the body that normally would occur in bone marrow.

"We knew that if Alex relapsed, he'd need a bone marrow transplant. His brothers rallied and gave what support they could by being there for Alex during his new chemo program to prep him for the procedure," Ellen said. When they learned Alex and Ellen would have to travel to Minneapolis for the transplant, they expressed concern that their mother wouldn't be around and that they would not be able to see Alex regularly.

"But they knew it was important, that our choices were limited, and that Alex didn't stand a chance of surviving if he didn't go where this treatment was available," Ellen added.

"Alex's doctors were ahead of the game in that they had already completed a bone marrow transplant search through the American Bone Marrow Donor

Registry. The registry is one of two that list possible bone marrow donors nationwide. The results indicated that Alex had a substantial number of potential matches available from unrelated donors in case he did relapse.

"We were all comforted by this information, especially since none of Alex's three brothers had matched him. Alex and I drove to Minneapolis, Minnesota, where the bone marrow transplant would take place. There, we met with a bone marrow transplant specialist and a bone marrow doctor.

"We talked about the procedure and the risks involved, which were many and worrisome. Alex could develop toxicity from his preparative regime, which could include serious complications in his liver, lungs, or heart. Massive internal bleeding was another risk, because Alex's red blood count was low. Mouth sores and loss of hair were two other side effects of the transplant, but we already were accustomed to dealing with those.

"Infection was a constant threat to Alex, and the bone marrow transplant procedure increased his vulnerability. And, of course, there was a chance the bone marrow graft would fail if Alex's body rejected it or if the new cells refused to grow. Add to that list graft-versus-host disease, relapse, and other complications, and you can see why this procedure caused us much concern.

"We also discussed what we could expect in terms of donor availability. We talked about expectations. We talked about the next round of chemo Alex would receive when we returned home, and what, if any, maintenance chemo would be required before the transplant.

"All that discussion didn't prepare us for the reality of the process. First, Alex had to endure nine days of chemo treatment that were straight from hell.

"Alex handled the first few days okay, and was transferred into the pediatric intensive care unit, partially in consideration of possible side effects. He couldn't eat. He had developed sores in the back of his throat and down his esophagus. He was on morphine for pain management—the side effects were worse than Alex had ever experienced. His nails were discolored. He developed severe diarrhea and began bleeding through his intestines. He asked me if he was going to die and I looked him straight in the eyes and told him that if we couldn't get his blood pressure to stabilize, he might.

"All together, Alex was in intensive care for three weeks before he rebounded, and he stayed in the Minneapolis hospital for a total of twenty-eight days. He started losing his skin, all of it. The effect was almost as if he had been burned from the inside out. He was disgusted—the skin on his hands was green. The heels of his feet came off in one piece. But Alex was still able to laugh. He wasn't feeling his greatest, but he had made it. We could go home and wait for the bone marrow transplant to be scheduled."

Alex's Quick Recovery from the Bone Marrow Transplant

Alex's mother explained that before Alex could have a bone marrow transplant, he had to have extensive dental work done on his mouth to prevent infection. Alex had already experienced infections so this was of particular concern to the doctors.

A surgeon removed several of Alex's teeth and part of his jawbone, which had died because of the infection and sores he had developed after the previous round of chemotherapy. This preventative dental work is fairly common when preparing cancer patients for invasive treatments such as bone marrow transplants. You could compare it to astronauts having their appendixes removed prior to prolonged space flights to avoid any medical emergencies.

Infection during a transplant is more dangerous than during chemo. Alex would be waiting for his white blood cells, and those of the donor's to return, meaning that the immune system is in a precarious state during a bone marrow transplant. Anything that could be done to prevent infection was done prior to the procedure.

Before such a transplant occurs, it is common for the patient to undergo yet another round of chemotherapy as well as total body irradiation. Transplant patients expect their blood counts to come back between thirty and thirty-four days after the procedure, and some as early as twenty-one days. Amazingly for Alex, his white blood cell count was back after only fourteen days.

Looking back at the overall experience, Alex's mother expressed her feelings about the chemotherapy sessions Alex underwent in his fight against leukemia: "In those two years, I watched as Alex faced the worst kind of chemotherapy. Those treatments were harsh enough to make me wonder if I could have tolerated them as well as he did."

Matt and His Family Face Chemotherapy: Another Perspective

As Told by His Mother, Sheri

"In addition to having a brain tumor surgically removed when he was two years old, Matt underwent chemotherapy. Like Alex, Matt had a central line in his chest, attached to an artery, to make giving him medications and nutrients easier and less painful.

"No one knows why people of all ages contract cancer, including brain tumors such as Matt's. It can occur in infants under the age of one year all the way to people in their eighties or nineties. Chemotherapy can be used to combat these cancers at any age, with the dosages and treatment cycles carefully monitored by oncologists.

"Matt had both inpatient and outpatient chemo sessions. Most of Matt's chemo was done in the hospital. However, he received one chemo drug called vincristine in our home at two different times during a chemo cycle. The Vincristine was administered as an IV push through Matt's central line.

"What this means is that the Vincristine was drawn into a syringe at the home health infusion company. The home health nurse, a specialist certified in chemotherapy, brought the filled syringe to our house and slowly injected the Vincristine into Matt's central line.

"As far as we could tell, Matt didn't feel a thing when this procedure was taking place. There were no pokes from needles because the syringe needle went into a special 'port', or opening, in the end of

the central line, so it was painless. Matt may have experienced a 'rush' or burning sensation, as the nurse told us many drugs administered by IV push can be felt in that way. But Matt was too young to tell us if this happened.

"We didn't have any oral chemo (drugs taken through the mouth as opposed to injected or pushed through an IV drip) at home as many leukemia patients do. Perhaps it was because of his age (twenty-two to forty-six months) or maybe because Matt's chemo drugs weren't available in oral form. Probably it wasn't a good way to give Matt chemo drugs anyway because he wouldn't have been able to swallow them."

The American Cancer Society confirms what Sheri believes—that prescribing oral chemo for Matt wouldn't have been a good idea. The society reports that some chemo drugs are never taken by mouth because the digestive system cannot absorb them, or because they irritate the digestive system. Even when a drug is available in oral form, using it may not be the best choice for patients like Matt, who already have diarrhea from continuous use of antibiotics or who cannot swallow pills safely.

"If Matt had had oral chemo, it would have gone through his g-tube [gastrostomy tube]. A g-tube was surgically implanted in Matt's stomach so we could feed him. It is sometimes called a button because it is a little stem about a half-inch long with a snap cap on it that looks much like a beach ball closure.

"When Matt's g-tube was used, the cap was opened and a short piece of tubing was placed on the button with an adapter. The tubing was hooked up to a bag of formula, wich looked very similar to an IV bag of saline solution The tubing went through a pump, which regulated how fast the formula flowed and how much Matt was fed. It was really quite simple. When we were not using the g-tube, the button covering was snapped shut. It sat nearly flush with Matt's skin, making a slight bump under his shirt.

"Matt needed the g-tube because his swallow, cough, and gag reflexes were damaged from the surgical procedure to remove the tumor. With those reflexes damaged, Matt was unable to eat by mouth. He did not have a protective airway, as the doctors termed it, which made it dangerous for him to eat by mouth. He could easily choke or have food go down the wrong way.

"Matt's tumor was at the base of his brain stem, right where all his vital functions are controlled. Within a year his nerves eventually recovered, and we no longer needed the g-tube. It was removed and the site on his stomach closed naturally.

"Matt's inpatient chemo sessions occurred during his first six months of treatment and were easier in some ways. We were admitted to one of our usual two rooms. We had one of the same two or three nurses every time, and at least we knew what to expect. Matt's first six months of chemotherapy were scheduled with a five-day inpatient stay at the hospital every twenty-one days. Within a few days of getting home from those hospital stays, we would end up back at the hospital because of infections, respiratory problems, the need for transfusions, and *other reasons. In fact, we were in the hospital more than we were home.*

"With these sessions completed, Matt was started on maintenance chemo. The schedule changed to a forty-nine-day cycle with two days of inpatient treatment. These treatments were still intense, but not as hard on him as the first series. And Matt was frequently hospitalized for infections and other problems that go along with chemo treatments."

The American Cancer Society says maintenance chemotherapy aims at three goals:

A. The first goal is to cure the cancer, meaning the tumor or cancer disappears and does not return. Smaller doses of chemo drugs are given to maintain an environment within the body that prevents cancer from flourishing or returning. This is the reason Matt was put on maintenance.

B. If it is not possible to cure the cancer, the second goal is to control it—to stop the disease from spreading and growing. This is done to help improve the quality of life for the cancer patient.

C. Sometimes cure and control are not possible if the cancer is in an advanced stage. At this point, the goal of maintenance chemo is palliation, which means the drugs will be used to relieve symptoms caused by the cancer. This will improve the quality of the patient's life, but will probably not prolong it.

"Many of those problems stemmed from neurological complications, which affected the things Matt couldn't do after surgery but could do before. The complications affected his ability to walk, talk, eat, use his hands, lift his head, and sit up. This caused further developmental delays because he could not access his environment the way he could prior to the surgery. He became very frustrated, making bad behavior somewhat an issue," said Sherri.

"These problems were not directly related to chemotherapy, but to by-products of it. Matt wasn't able to play or move about as a normal two-year-old would be expected. His doctor said his development just plain stopped during treatment because he was too sick to play, interact with others, and simply be a kid.

"We also ran into some pulmonary problems with Matt. The chemo caused a disease in his lungs—interstitial lung disease, which is rare but documented. This required breathing support and a continuous supply of oxygen. The treatment for this disease involved steroids, bringing a whole new set of complications to bear on Matt's situation.

"Steroids affect the immune system, and Matt's system was already dangerously compromised from the chemotherapy. It took coordination between the pulmonary and oncology staff to make sure that what one person gave him interacted in the right way with whatever else was being given. It was a very scary time for us. Matt's lung disease had been resolved but his obstructive airway was still a problem.

"The obstructive airway problem was caused by paralyzed vocal chords, and it in turn created problems with managing Matt's breathing. That is why we needed to have a tracheotomy implanted in Matt one week after his surgery.

"The trach and g-tube were additional sites that harbored bacteria, causing infections easily because Matt was so immune-suppressed from the chemo. Most cancer patients don't have these problems. They usually have to deal only with the typical bloodstream infections caused by low blood counts. But Matt was generally on some IV antibiotic the whole time to prevent these infections. That in turn caused other problems such as diarrhea.

"Matt never experienced the classic nausea and vomiting associated with chemotherapy. He coped by watching Winnie the Pooh and Barney videos. He could hardly hold a toy, much less play with it. During this period, he was functioning more like a six- to nine-month-old instead of a two-year-old. Most of his inpatient and outpatient chemo treatments were spent in front of the VCR.

"Radiation was never used on Matt. The medical protocols that govern cancer treatment stress that radiation therapy should not be used on patients under the age of three. Therapists are concerned about severe damage that can occur to the undeveloped brain of a very young child. Matt's chemotherapy protocol was an eighteen-month course, but it really took about twenty months to complete because of delays from infections and sepsis, a form of blood poisoning."

Through all the months of treatment, Sheri and Matt's father, Greg, plus Matt's older brother, Joey, faced many day-to-day upsets and setbacks. Matt was *frustrated and irritable because he couldn't play or do the things he had done before surgery. He frequently cried, fretted, and generally behaved badly. This is a normal reaction in most cancer patients who get tired of dealing with pain and feeling helpless, regardless of their age.*

Sheri cried, too. But her tears were a way of releasing the tension of caring for Matt through all the bewildering changes and complicated medical treatments, plus all her fears and worries for her fragile son. What made it more difficult for Sheri was that Matt couldn't tell her what was wrong or bothering him. Because of the surgery, Matt couldn't talk for many months.

Young Joey, just four years old when his brother Matt was diagnosed with brain stem cancer, sometimes seemed to be resentful of how his home life had been disrupted.

The family relied on the strength and support of family and friends through this ordeal. Someone was always there when Sheri needed help. The doctors and nurses who helped treat Matt became staunch helpers as well, answering Sheri's and Greg's many questions patiently and honestly.

As you have read, chemotherapy and the other methods used to combat cancer can seem nearly as bad as suffering from the disease. And it doesn't help that each person reacts differently. Side effects depend partially on what type of cancer the patient is fighting, what kinds and combination of chemo drugs are prescribed, and how long the treatments last. But most important, they depend on the individual.

Experts have found no way to predict how any one person will react to chemo or radiation therapy. Almost every cancer patient experiences one or more of the common side effects during treatment, and it's not unusual for some side effects to continue afterward. Because no statistical averages exist to help you prepare mentally for what might happen to your family member, the best thing you can do is take each day as it comes and deal with side effects on a one-at-a-time basis.

Now that you know these side effects can and often do occur, it will help you cope with them if or when they occur in your family member. Here are some suggestions:

A. "Don't sweat the small stuff" is a useful slogan to keep in mind. Hair loss, discolored fingernails, weight loss or gain, and other physical changes may not seem small to you, but they are in relationship to what chemotherapy and radiation therapy can do to help your loved one survive cancer. Look past these superficial changes in your family member as much as possible. The parent, brother, or sister you love is still the same person underneath it all.

B. Accept the fact that your family member is critically ill. Sometimes, this is hard to do because then you have to face all the possibilities that go with a cancer diagnosis. You may be tempted to shut out the cancer, but if you do, you also shut out your loved one. Once you accept the diagnosis, it will change your perspective about harsh side effects such as vomiting, nausea, and diarrhea.

C. Do what you can when you can to help distract the patient. This may not seem like much, but just being there for the patient can make a huge difference in how he or she gets through the side effects' discomfort. Playing games, listening to music, watching television, or doing your favorite things together all can help take the patient's mind off his or her condition.

D. Try to keep things as normal as possible. This is the tough one because obviously things are not going to be "normal" in your home. Often, the patient will be hospitalized. During those times, sticking to your regular routine as much as you can will help you feel in control and balanced. When the patient is home, make an effort to do exactly what the two of you did before the cancer diagnosis. If that's not possible because of the patient's condition, try to establish a new routine that accommodates both your needs and the patient's ability to join in.

The best advice families of cancer patients offer is to take each day as it comes. Remember that the chosen therapy and its side effects are temporary for the most part. This will help you hold on to a positive, optimistic outlook.

The Cancer Patient at Home: Changes Will Be Made

For a cancer patient to be treated successfully at home, many changes will have to be made, says Patty Kirkham, the oncology social worker for Rockford Health Services.

She adds, "It's important to accept what is happening in your family and then to make adjustments. People grieve the loss of normalcy. That's natural. It may feel as if your whole world has been turned upside down, but when that happens, it helps to know that the patient is grieving the loss of normal life as well. Working toward acceptance together is far better than remaining separate from the issues."

These changes might include trading your first-floor bedroom for one upstairs or for a bedroom in the basement, so that your brother or sister is more accessible to your parents and in-home treatment. Or, the living or dining room may suddenly be transformed into a hospital room, filled with a dismaying array of medical equipment and supplies.

Food

Having a cancer patient at home may also mean major changes in the kinds of foods that are in your house. Cancer patients often don't feel like eating. Or, sometimes, he or she may be able to eat only specific foods and nothing else. At other times, depending on the type of cancer your family member has, a special diet may need to be followed. You might be expected to eat the same foods. On the other hand, you might find yourself eating a lot more fast food, such as pizza or hamburgers, because your mother, father, or other relative doesn't have time to cook.

Free Time
Having a seriously ill sibling or parent in your home will probably change the way you spend your free time. Don't be surprised if there are new restrictions on the amount of noise you're allowed to make and the number of friends you can invite over. Cancer patients must be protected from fresh sources of infection. They need a peaceful atmosphere and a lot of rest in order to help them heal.

Financial Security
Catastrophic illnesses such as cancer often affect a family's financial resources. This could mean that there is less money for new clothes, family vacations, involvement in extracurricular activities at school, and other things you've taken for granted before.

How Will We Pay for This?

Among the secondary questions families face after a cancer diagnosis is, "How will we pay for this?" Costs vary depending on the type of treatment, how long and how often it is given, and whether the patient is treated at home, in a hospital, or in a clinic or doctor's office. Your family will need to find out what your health insurance plan, Medicare Part B, or Medicaid will pay for before deciding on a treatment plan.

Health insurance will cover part of the cost to treating your family member, but no insurance policy covers all of it. And sometimes, people do not have health insurance at all. This is a serious problem because the cost of treating cancer can amount to hundreds of thousands of dollars.

One of the first things your parents should do is check the patient's eligibility for state or local benefits such as Medicaid. This is helpful if your family falls into the middle- or low-income bracket, or if one of your parents is unemployed. If a parent is planning to quit working to care for the patient, he or she may want to discuss insurance conversion plans.

If your parents are looking at insurance options, they need to be aware of the differences in coverage. They should ask about choosing doctors, protection against policy cancellation, and unexpected increases in premiums. Your parents need to know exactly what each plan actually covers, especially for catastrophic illnesses such as cancer. Deductibles are another factor that will help your parents determine which plan to buy because some plans with higher deductibles (the part your family pays) cover more of the costs than plans with lower deductibles.

Some insurance plans pay for medical trials and the most advanced cancer treatments, while others will pay only for the "tried and true" treatments. Others limit what treatments they will pay for, and will determine which hospitals, clinics, and doctors the patient may use. This can be extremely frustrating when you're dealing with the survival of a loved one.

"We had an insurance plan that covered things such as durable medical equipment—e.g., wheelchairs, hospital beds—at 100 percent," Matt's mother, Sheri, said. "That's very unusual because most plans cover this at 80 percent, with the policyholder paying the other 20 percent."

Sheri said Matt's hospitalization was also covered 100 percent with a copay of $100. All of his outpatient visits were covered 100 percent with a $10 copay. Emergency room charges were $50 with 100 percent covered after that. All of Matt's home health nursing and related services, including equipment, drugs, and therapy were negotiated out of their own service network by their HMO, so they also cost Matt's family nothing.

"Our insurance company was painfully slow in paying bills. Many went to collection agencies," Sheri added. "But we eventually got them straightened out."

This was a good thing, Sheri said, because Matt's medical expenses were "staggering." At one time, the family was notified that his hospital bill was down to $500,000! That didn't include doctors' bills, radiology, laboratory, MRI readings, anesthesiology, home health service, therapy, home infusions of chemo drugs, home equipment, infection, lung disease treatments, and more.

"We didn't receive detailed invoices, so we just hoped they'd get paid," Sheri said. "At that time, I didn't even open our mail for at least six months or so—I was just too overwhelmed to handle it."

Another important aspect of insurance that Sheri mentioned is that, no matter how good or bad an insurance company is, someone in your family will have to spend a tremendous amount of time on the telephone with them—mostly on hold.

"You need a lot of patience, not to mention anger control, in dealing with insurance companies," Sheri added. "There you sit, hoping your child lives through the day, trying to talk to some uninformed person doing his or her best to save money for the insurance company. It can be frustrating and heartbreaking."

Ellen faced challenges in dealing with Alex's insurance coverage as well. "I was covered by COBRA at work when Alex was diagnosed," Ellen explained. "It was good until my former employer decided to drop us in June 1999. When I called to ask why we weren't being given more than nine days' notice, I was told 'what's the point?'"

Alex's initial chemotherapy and hospitalization were covered at about 90 percent. His bone marrow transplant had been prequalified with the insurance company and was covered 100 percent. Ellen's insurance company had a contract under the United Resources Network, as do a number of other health plans, for exactly that purpose. It was this plan that determined where Alex would receive his bone marrow treatment.

In addition, Alex qualified for Medicaid, which picked up the bill on the bone marrow transplant procedure. Ellen had applied for Alex immediately after he relapsed in July 1998. As required before his transplant, Alex had made a living will, which told the doctors to what extent he wanted to be revived in case of a serious medical setback.

"For many families, there is a lack of recognition when a child goes from sixteen or seventeen to legal adult status," Ellen said. "That brings in a whole world of different considerations, including whether doctors will still allow parents the same input now that the child is legally an adult and can make his or her own decisions."

Ellen stressed how important the insurance aspect is to families of cancer patients. So many companies are trying to limit what they cover and what they won't, she explained. They are trying to determine what is needed in a situation where only a doctor and the patient have the right to make choices regarding treatment and care.

"There are some children who have never had local anesthesia for a bone marrow biopsy because of their insurance," Ellen added. "Without the local, kids experience a lot of pain. Alex did that once, with Novocaine as the only pain blocker. It was miserable."

Caring for Alex and Matt at Home

Here's what happened in Alex's and Matt's homes while they were being treated for their cancers.

Between hospitalizations and inpatient treatments, Alex received a tremendous amount of care at home. His mother, Ellen, was responsible for the greater part of that care. And, as you read in past chapters, his brothers also contributed in different ways. This is how Ellen recalls that experience.

"My husband, Roy, and I were separated at the time Alex was diagnosed with leukemia," Ellen said. "Roy moved back home to be near seventeen-year-old Alex.

"Meanwhile, I had been working full-time. I chose to work fewer hours so I could be home to take care of Alex. I had to learn how to inject medications such as insulin for his steroid-induced diabetes. GCSF [granulocyte colony stimulating factor], which encouraged the growth of neutrophils [white blood cells found in the bone marrow of the spine], antibiotics, which prevented and fought infections, and even preparatory medications used to knock Alex out for painful procedures. All of these procedures were given through his central line. Each medication necessitated a particular procedure for flushing the line.

"I learned how to change Alex's central line dressings and to do many other things I had never even thought about needing to know how to do. I was scared to death. I spent most of the first three weeks crying nightly and trying to analyze whether I was being overprotective or whether I was not doing enough. Alex never commented on this.

"Because Alex's leukemia made him vulnerable to infection, all of us, including Forrest, Danny, and Lucas, were careful to wash our hands before we undertook any kind of care that involved touching Alex.

"Despite the struggle he had getting up the stairs after his first chemotherapy session, Alex kept his room on the second floor. It became his refuge. At first, the family made only small changes to the house—a hook in Alex's room on which to hang his IV and medication bags, a bedside commode *for the times he couldn't get to the bathroom quickly enough. Our home also became a supply depot for all the things we needed to care for him properly: bandages, syringes, medications, normal saline solution, paper tape, IV tubing.*

"But after Alex came home from his bone marrow transplant, things around the house began to change more noticeably. Because of his more fragile condition, we didn't dare leave him alone. Someone always had to be there for him. Later, when Alex was unable to get around by himself, I requested a wheelchair, which he used until his final hospitalization.

"When he began to need more IV medication, we added a Sabretek ambulatory IV pump and pole. The pump ensures that saline solution and medications flow smoothly in the proper direction. By using this equipment, we were able to move Alex around the house as needed.

"Getting Alex in and out of the house was only slightly problematic. But lifting him in and out of the van when the family went out was a challenge. We developed a 'left, right' rhythm, which Alex remembered and used just as he used cues he learned from his physical therapist to help him get out of bed and into his wheelchair. Because Alex was in a wheelchair, he was unable to fix his own meals, so they were prepared for him. Keeping him in good health and at an appropriate weight was extremely important.

"When Alex was diagnosed as a steroid-induced diabetic [a condition that can occur when any cancer patient is taking prednisone or other chemo-related

steroid drugs], meals became an occupation in themselves, along with administering all his medications and checking his glucose levels.

"Alex's diet was determined by the hospital's nutritionist, then modified by his endocrinologist, a specialist who works with glands that secrete fluids into the bloodstream. With Alex, the endocrinologist focused on the pancreas, where insulin is normally manufactured.

"Blood for the tests needed to monitor Alex's glucose levels was taken from his central line, avoiding the need to repeatedly stick his fingers with needles four times a day. This way, his fingertips didn't become sore and extremely sensitive as is the case with most diabetics."

At this point, Ellen said Alex's brothers didn't react in an obvious way to the news that their brother was diabetic. Instead, they seemed to have adopted a "what next" attitude.

Alex told Ellen that, once the central line was put in, he firmly believed everyone should have one because it alleviates being stuck with needles.

"Alex's physical condition continued to decline, and we gave up the struggle of trying to get him up and down the stairs. It was just too risky. We had a hospital bed brought in and placed in the living room. Whenever his brothers had company, they had to keep in mind that this was now Alex's room. They were asked to be quiet and courteous if Alex was resting or sleeping. When Alex's white blood cell count was too low and danger of infection was high, visits to our home were restricted in order to protect him."

The boys understood and accepted this well, Ellen said. They knew how delicate Alex's immune system was after seeing him suffer through so many infections. Not only did they comply with the restrictions to visits from their friends at home, they didn't push for visiting Alex whenever he was hospitalized for infections.

On the other hand, when they were able to visit Alex, they planned on staying with him as much as possible, including overnight, Ellen added. When they couldn't see him, they called a lot. And when Alex was far away for the bone marrow transplant in Minneapolis, they e-mailed him almost daily.

During this time, Alex's brothers received no counseling even though it was available through the hospital. Instead, Ellen talked to them constantly and tried to keep them informed on Alex's condition in an honest, straightforward manner.

"My suggestion is to talk openly to each other. It's a fact of life for cancer patients. The best thing is to meet it all head-on," Ellen added. "If anyone in your family is having problems facing the situation, then seeking counseling becomes much more important.

"You can ask the oncologists and other specialists treating your family member as well," Ellen said. "My sons had a great rapport with every one of Alex's doctors. If they felt the need to ask something, they knew they could. They accepted that the doctors were accountable to them, too, up to a point."

Matt was not discharged from the hospital until two months after his surgery for a brain tumor. But once Matt did come home, twenty-four-hour nursing care was a necessity. Matt's mother, Sheri, explains how they coped.

"Because Matt needed twenty-four-hour care, we had to deal with a ton of paperwork from the hospital each time we brought him home. It also meant that we had to deal with what seemed like hundreds of telephone calls clarifying orders and giving reports to Matt's doctor, plus running to the drugstore for medicines.

"Hardly a day went by without us receiving deliveries—some of which were bewildering—that were vital to Matt's total home care. Just to name a few, we received a ventilator, pulse oximeter, and oxygen concentrator as well as an oxygen humidity system to aid Matt's breathing. We had IV poles, feeding bags, and tubing, plus TPN and kangaroo pumps for feeding Matt. We had a wheelchair, and a hospital crib and bed. We needed a suction machine, sterile and nonsterile gloves, tracheotomy supplies, sterile gauze for dressings, sterile water, sterile saline, and heparin to flush Matt's central line. We received boxes of syringes and biohazard bags.

"That was just a partial list of what seemed like tons of stuff. Fortunately, our HMO covered all of this 100 percent. It all came to our house in one way or another, without our going to a pharmacy or home health care store to pick it up. It was all considered either medical supplies or durable medical equipment and was covered. Our insurance coverage was great—and still is.

"Our dining room was immediately converted to a hospital room in order to accommodate the care Matt needed. The home health equipment company set us up with a hospital crib, a ventilator, a suction machine, a breathing machine, an oxygen system and IV pole to handle the humidifier system, an IV pole to hang his feeding bags, pumps to run the IVs, and shelves upon shelves of other medical necessities.

"I soon become very familiar with the sight of syringes, lab specimen containers, tape, tubing, cases of pediatric formula, boxes of diapers, cases of suctioning catheters, and dozens more items stacked around the dining room. Those items that didn't fit into the dining room were stored in the sunroom nearby. I could never have believed that we would ever need or use all those things, but trust me, we used all those things and more.

"Home stays were sometimes barely twenty-four hours long. Matt's condition would deteriorate to the point where he had to return to the hospital where doctors would treat the awful effects of chemotherapy, along with infections and other problems. Many times we had not even unpacked our bags before we were repacking to go back to the hospital. The situation was so difficult that family members who lived far away actually came to help out. Eventually, the running of our household was more or less turned over to our mothers and other relatives. They took turns and stayed at our house for a week or so each."

Matt's mother committed herself to helping the nurse take care of Matt because he was a two-person *responsibility. Matt's father, Greg, returned to work on a modified schedule. His older brother Joey, then four years old, continued to attend his all-day pre-kindergarten because his parents felt that would be the best thing for him to do. "It also freed us of the distraction of trying to care for both Joey and Matt. When I gave birth to our baby daughter, the role of our parents and families became an even greater one. They took care of our newborn and Joey, while we worked to save Matt's life."*

Helping and Asking for Help

As you have read, the changes in Alex's home started out as minor ones and grew steadily as his need for more intensive care increased. On the other hand, Matt's home was turned topsy-turvy from the moment he came home from the hospital.

There is no way to accurately predict what will happen in any family when one of its members is diagnosed with cancer. So much depends on the type of cancer, the family member who is diagnosed, the methods of treatment, whether the treatment is close to home or far away, and more. However, one thing is certain: Changes will occur. Learning to deal effectively with the changes instead of fighting them will help you and your family get through the difficult times.

For example, you might have to give up your bedroom or share a bedroom with another sibling while the patient is at home recovering from treatment. You probably won't be able to avoid these kinds of situations. But while you might have to give up some things, you shouldn't feel as if you have to give up everything. For example, if you continue to participate in extracurricular activities at school and one of your parents usually picks you up afterward, you can ask one of your classmates to let you share his or her ride home instead of giving up the activity. The same holds true if you want to visit a parent or sibling in the hospital and you need someone else to drive you there.

In fact, you can ask for help from a lot of people from whom you wouldn't usually expect to receive it. You'll find that people in your school, neighborhood, and community will want to help. But because they're not family members, they may not know what kind of help to offer until you or a family member asks.

Don't automatically say no when someone asks if he or she can help. Most of us are not used to needing help from people outside our immediate family. During the time your family member is undergoing treatment, you might become so deeply involved that you may not even realize that you need help. Or, like so many independent people, you might not know how to say yes, or how to ask for some assistance.

On the Pediatric Oncology Resource Center's Web site, one family member of a cancer patient commented that what most people forget is that coping with cancer in the family is a long-term family problem. Help with meals and other things the first few weeks after diagnosis are wonderful, but the family is looking at dealing with this situation for a year or longer. It's easy for people to fade from the picture, but emotional support is crucial. So, even if you don't have a specific chore for the helper to perform, just being there for you when you need someone is plenty.

So, say yes to offers of help, even if you're not sure at the time exactly what kind of help you'll need. Ask friends, neighbors, and relatives to call on a regular basis. And when they do, don't hesitate to tell them what you need.

Reaching Out to Family, Friends, and Support Groups

When someone in your family is first diagnosed with cancer, you may feel as if your whole family has suddenly been left to drift alone on a dark and dangerous sea. No matter what kinds of emotions you are dealing with, and no matter how hard this time may be, it is important to remember that support is available.

Usually, close family members and/or friends are the first to respond to your family's crisis. Those who live close by may come daily to help, while those who live further away may come to visit or may frequently express emotional support from a distance. You might be asked to stay with other family members from time to time while your parents focus on helping whichever family member is ill.

In your community, there may be support groups based at local hospitals, colleges, or health clinics. These groups are comprised of patients and/or family members who are also coping with cancer. They are usually led by medical professionals such as doctors, oncology specialists, and oncology social workers. Through these groups, you can connect with other teens who are facing the same things that you are. To find out more about these groups, contact your hospital's supportive services office. If the hospital in which your family member is being treated does not have a teen support group, the staff oncology social worker may be able to help you find one in a hospital nearby.

Some hospital and clinic systems offer a program called Ask a Nurse. By calling this organization, you can talk to a registered nurse who can answer general questions about support groups. Hospitals may also offer automatic response services that are listed in a brochure or in the front of your local telephone directory. To access this service, you dial one telephone number, then dial a four- or five-digit number that automatically connects you to a prerecorded message concerning the subject you've requested.

Your community may also have local chapters affiliated with national organizations such as the American Cancer Society, CanTeen, or Candlelighters International. Through associations such as these, you will find a wealth of information and advice, plus the different kinds of support you may need as the treatment of your family member progresses. You'll find a list of some possibilities in the back of this book. And you will be able to find more in your local telephone book as well.

The Internet can also provide a lot of unlimited supportive assistance—ranging from information about the different kinds of cancer to inspirational stories to chat rooms and e-mail subscription resources. However, you should know that you need to be careful when dealing with information on the Internet. Some of the sites may not be accurate. You'll find reliable Web addresses listed in the Where to Go for Help section in the back of this book.

Unfortunately, it would be impossible to list in this book all the available resources for people who are coping with cancer in their families. But once you begin to search, you'll find links that will help you focus in on exactly what you need and provide answers to your questions.

Alex's Support Network

When Alex was first diagnosed with leukemia, the regional chapter of Candlelighters had not yet been organized. According to Alex's mother, "There were people who knew other families in the same situation, but nothing was organized. Alex and I met a couple of the kids and their parents, and got to know them. But we had no direct contact with any national organizations other than research I did through them on the Internet."

"The hospital staff on the pediatrics floor where Alex was being treated became the family's greatest source of support. I felt I could talk to them on the level I needed about Alex's medical condition and his needs," Ellen explained. "The rest of my family depended on me to ask the appropriate questions and get the answers for them.

"Seeing his football team play was important to Alex. Many of his teammates visited him in the hospital right after his diagnosis, including the player who had tackled Alex during practice. Alex's friends buoyed his spirits and kept him in touch with what was going on in school. They visited only on occasion, not wanting to compromise his weakened immune system.

"The varsity football team dedicated its season to Alex. One teammate ordered wristbands made with Alex's number on them and received permission for the team to wear them during games as a show of support. This meant a lot, not just to Alex but to his entire family.

"A number of people started fund-raising drives for Alex that fall. My best friend and her family had a benefit which included a band. A junior at Alex's high school started selling ribbons featuring the school colors with Alex's name on them. She later added teddy bears to her collection to sell. And a group of Alex's classmates donated money from a bowl-a-thon.

"The mothers of Alex's classmates were preparing meals and bringing them to the house whenever they could," Ellen continued. Because Ellen was still working part-time and spending increasing amounts of time with Alex in the hospital, she was often too exhausted to do much at home.

"Their generosity was overwhelming to Alex and the rest of us," Ellen added. "We were very grateful."

Make-A-Wish Foundation and Ronald McDonald House Charities

Just about the time Alex was going into remission from his leukemia, he and his family met with a representative from the Make-A-Wish Foundation. This nonprofit organization grants wishes to children under age eighteen who are facing life-threatening illnesses.

The Make-A-Wish Foundation grants requests from any of several potential referral sources, including the child, parents or legal guardians, and the medical professional treating the child such as his or her doctor, social worker, or child life specialist.

After receiving the referral, the foundation determines eligibility, based on the age of the child. The child's doctor makes the final decision on whether he or she is medically eligible to receive a wish and whether or not he or she can participate in the wish. The child must be able to talk about the wish and cannot have had a wish granted through another agency. Also, the child must be a legal citizen of the United States or live in a country served by an international affiliate.

The next step is to identify the wish. The foundation assigns a volunteer wish team to coordinate the wish-granting process. When the team first visits the child, the volunteers ask one simple question: "If you could have one wish, what would it be?" Usually, wishes are limited only by the child's imagination. Most wishes fall into one of four groups: "I want to go . . ."; "I want to be . . ."; "I want to meet . . ."; or "I want to have . . ." Once the local chapter approves the wish, the team sets out to make it come true.

After talking to the patient, the Make-A-Wish team creates a magical wish experience for the child that will be remembered for a lifetime. The wish experience often touches dozens, even hundreds of people who either help coordinate or are directly involved in the wish.

The Make-A-Wish experiences granted by the foundation's eighty chapters are made possible through the support of thousands of corporate and private donors, as well as a pool of more than 18,000 volunteers nationwide.

Alex just qualified agewise, Ellen said. His wish? To go to Seattle. Why? Alex couldn't say for sure, he just knew that he'd always wanted to go there. So, in February 1998, Alex and his entire family flew to Seattle. The Make-A-Wish Foundation had granted Alex's wish. Seattle in February is usually cold and rainy, but while Alex and his family were there, there was little rain, and the weather was beautiful.

"For anyone not acquainted with this organization, it's a godsend," Ellen said. "The trip was planned not just for Alex but for his family, with everything paid for by Make-A-Wish, including spending money for the boys. The only worry we had was whether we'd be able to eat all the meals in the schedule."

Alex's family stayed at the Edgewater Hotel, the only hotel on the water in downtown Seattle. They dined atop the Space Needle, visited the architects and the construction site of the new baseball stadium, went to the zoo, and ate at Planet Hollywood. The trip included tickets to a Sonics-Celtics basketball game, and Alex was invited to listen in at the Celtic's pregame session. Player Vin Baker presented Alex with his game shoes, complete with sweat and autograph.

"We had a great time, and we brought home wonderful memories," Ellen added.

The Make-A-Wish Foundation wasn't the only organization that brightened those dark days for Alex and his family. While Alex and Ellen were in Minneapolis for his bone marrow transplant in December 1998, Alex's swift recovery resulted in his being released to the Ronald McDonald House on Christmas Eve.

"Alex's early release wasn't the only surprise," Ellen said. "We had expected his father and brothers to arrive Christmas morning for a two-day visit. We had no sooner arrived at Ronald McDonald House and gotten Alex comfortable than the phone rang." Alex's dad and brothers had arrived early, and he was thrilled, Ellen recalled.

"Christmas morning arrived, and so did gifts from Santa," Ellen added. "The generosity of Ronald McDonald House was just beginning to become apparent."

Outside the door of the family's two-room suite was a bag filled with gifts for the boys. Alex's dad and brothers had brought gifts they'd purchased plus those from the rest of the family. But the best gift, Ellen stressed, was that they could all be together in a homelike setting. Alex's girlfriend drove to Minneapolis and stayed for two days. After she left, Alex's best friend and her family arrived to spend New Year's Day.

Ronald McDonald House Charities' global office provides each house with seed money, expansion and emergency grants, as well as in-kind goods and services. But it's up to the community in which the house is based to provide additional funding, goods, and services as needed for its operation. Alex's family had a lot to thank the people of Minneapolis for, as they celebrated the holidays far from home.

The entire Ronald McDonald House program is supported by nearly 25,000 volunteers who donate more than one million hours of their time each year to helping families such as Alex's. Families staying at Ronald

McDonald Houses are asked to make a donation ranging from $5 to $20 per day. But if that's not possible, their stay is free.

"The hospital offered a program called Care Partners," Ellen added. "Alex and I used this program. A local, caring individual is assigned to each family to help them out, run errands, and provide support. The person assigned was a transplant survivor who stayed with Alex and who watched movies or played games with Alex when I had to be away from him."

At home, Ellen and her family became part of a support group that consisted primarily of nurses and the father of one former patient who had died not long after Alex was diagnosed.

Matt's Support Network

When Matt was diagnosed with a brain tumor, the rest of his family rallied to the aid of Sheri and Greg.

"Everyone in our family was, of course, devastated and saddened," Sheri said. "However, all of our brothers and sisters, in-laws, and parents rose to the occasion in their own able ways." One brother drove the 100-plus miles from Chicago and spent many nights in the pediatric intensive care unit holding Matt's hand so that Sheri and Greg could go home and rest. One brother-in-law began donating blood at the local blood bank to help offset the tremendous need Matt would have for transfusions.

"My sisters rotated coming to stay for a few days, taking turns at the house or hospital. They also spent a lot of nights at the hospital because we needed

most to be there during the day. They brought meals to be stored in the freezer." Greg has a sister who lives close by and she became the family's first-line baby-sitter and errand runner. She also has two boys who became the only children to visit Matt in the hospital besides his older brother, Joey. The youngest, Scottie, began entertaining Matt in the most childlike, appropriate way no adult could match. This is where many of Matt's smiles came from. Matt's aunts also took brother Joey home to spend the night or weekend at their homes, giving him a break from the crisis and allowing him to resume a more normal pattern of living.

"It also gave us a much-needed break from trying to spend quality time with him and arranging baby-sitting while we went to and from the hospital. When we had our baby daughter, our families 'lived-in,' and they became her primary caregivers.

"Matt's grandparents spent time with him during hospital stays as well, but I think they were more comfortable at the hospital than at home with him. If something happened at the hospital, they were only a few feet away from the nurses' station. My parents' favorite thing to do was to prop Matt up in a wagon and wheel him around the hospital room, tethered to his oxygen system."

Candlelighters

Ellen and Sheri are members of the same regional Candlelighters organization for families of children diagnosed with cancer. Their group is the Rockford Area

Candlelighters in Illinois. Until a few years ago, the nationwide organization was funded by the American Cancer Society, but it was dropped from the society's budget. It is now self-funded.

Sheri said Rockford's chapter regrouped early in 1999 at the suggestion of one of the pediatric oncologists. The chapter meets monthly at the hospital. The meetings either are informal discussions that focus on a particular topic or feature a speaker. The group also plans at least one social get-together each month for the the members and their entire families.

"I am the president, and we have about thirty-five families listed within our group," Sheri added. "Some families have Angels, as we prefer to call those who could no longer fight their fight. Other families have children in treatment currently or who have completed treatment and are in remission or are cured."

As satisfying as her affiliation to Candlelighters is, Sheri said, she receives additional support from other on-line groups to which she and Greg subscribe: the Pediatric Oncology Resource Center and the medulloblastoma list (the particular brain cancer with which Matt was diagnosed), as well as the Candlelighters' e-mail list. You'll find these e-mail addresses in the Where to Go for Help section at the end of this book.

"The volume is heavy, up to sixty messages some days, but well worth the time spent on them," Sheri pointed out. "Perspectives, problems, and protocols from people all over the world are discussed. I would highly recommend this type of support system to anyone who has on-line access."

How to Give and Receive Support

In addition to finding the support you need personally to cope and stepping up your responsibilities at home to help your parents, there are some things you can ask friends and their parents to do to help lift the patient's morale.

If the patient is a sibling, you can ask the parents to carpool friends to the hospital for visits when it's appropriate. As Ellen and Sheri would tell you, having friends visit is a sure way to cheer up a hospitalized child. For teenage patients, staying in touch with friends and with what's happening at school is very important. If friends ask what they can do or give to make hospital treatments or those long hours at home easier to face, suggest that they give gift certificates for video rentals. Cassettes and CDs to play on a Walkman or Discman also alleviate the tedium and help distract the patient from what's happening to his or her body during treatments.

If the patient is a younger sibling, ask his or her friends to start a collection of favorite things, such as stickers or coloring books. This will give the patient something fun and positive to look forward to and do to pass the time. This way, those friends will know what to send or bring, when they might not know what else they can do to help.

Ask to spend more time with your friends at their homes when your sibling or parent is hospitalized. This will get you out of the house and into a more natural setting. This will also benefit your parents, who won't have to worry so much about not being there for you during those times when they have to be with the patient.

Let your friends know you'll need their support and understanding for a long time, not just the first few weeks or months after your family member is diagnosed with cancer. It's not unusual for parents and teens to lose some of their friends or to become distanced from relatives during this period.

Emotional support is as crucial to you as it is to every other member of your family. Ask your friends and relatives to call once or twice each week. Sometimes people don't know what to say, so they don't call. It might be necessary to remind them gently that you and your family have a life besides the cancer situation. You can do this by talking about school, hobbies, sports, movies, books, your healthy family members, or anything else you would have chatted about under more normal circumstances.

Coping with cancer when you are part of a single-parent family may be even more difficult. Your immediate family may consist of very few people, and they may not be close enough to help in any significant manner. Your school friends, neighbors, church or temple congregation, parent's friends and coworkers, as well as the hospital's support services are the people you can turn to for help. Even just a few people can make a tremendous difference in how you and your parent face this challenge.

There is no reason to "go it alone," and there is every reason to build a team of medical professionals, family, friends, and peers to help you through the tough times. Coping means facing this challenge in a positive manner.

Maintaining Your Balance: Attitude and Optimism

The adage "laughter is the best medicine" may be more than just an old saying. Many people, including an increasing number of medical professionals, are beginning to believe that humor and a strong, positive mental attitude are as important to overcoming cancer and other life-threatening illnesses as are treatments and drugs.

This theory applies not only to the patient, but to the caregivers and family as well. Sharing laughter, good memories, and an optimistic view of the future are vital elements of the recovery process. One reason is that depression is common during diagnosis and treatment of cancer, and it isn't just the patient who is vulnerable to it.

"Humor is essential in dealing with such a terrible disease," said Patty Kirkham, the oncology social worker. "I don't know what anyone would do without it. Whatever happens, keep your sense of humor intact."

As in the case of successful stand-up comedians, Patty added, timing is everything. "There is a time to laugh and a time to cry, but humor is an excellent way to get through those day-to-day situations where you feel you can either laugh or cry. When it's up to you to choose how you'll face the immediate problem, try to smile and lighten the pain."

As is true of so many other challenges in life, maintaining a positive attitude is crucial to how you cope when someone in your family has cancer.

How Alex and His Family Faced an Uncertain Future

After Alex's diagnosis, his mother, Ellen, asked Alex what he wanted her to do. He said that whenever he stopped fighting or didn't fight hard enough, she was to push him, prod him, motivate him, make him fight. His mother did that, right to the end.

Alex started making decisions and setting goals within days of being diagnosed with leukemia. His first goal was to be out of the hospital for his birthday, and then to attend the homecoming game at his high school. The second goal was to be home for Christmas and Thanksgiving. Alex's next goal was to go to the prom. But his last was the hardest to envision. Alex was determined to graduate with his senior class. His family was making goals in September for May, which might as well have been 40 million years in the future.

Despite intensive chemotherapy and a series of infections that kept Alex in the hospital for weeks at a time, he was home for both Thanksgiving and Christmas that year. Goal number two had been met.

Christmas took on a whole new meaning that year. No one knew what the next year might bring. The family was glad that they had made it so far, and that they were still together.

By the end of January, Alex was in remission from his leukemia. What he wanted most was to go back to school. Alex had tried working with a tutor, but between his chemotherapy and infections, he hadn't had a long enough span of good days to be productive. Fortunately, Alex had planned well for his high school years. To graduate, he needed only two more credits.

Most people would have been happy just to get back and get through those two, but not Alex. He needed to be in school for at least three periods daily, which would give him an extra credit. Why? Although it was a long shot, he wanted to try out for his varsity baseball team.

Alex went back to school on the first Monday in February 1998. While his schedule would be interrupted by doctor's appointments, Alex made the most of his days in class. During one visit to his oncologist, Alex told him he needed a pass to play sports in school. The doctor was hesitant, but Alex informed him that he'd play anyway. The note was just to make the school more comfortable. The next day, Alex took a note to school stating he could participate in all but contact sports. Alex was happy with that. Watching sports from the sideline was like cutting his arm off. He wanted to be active. And it was good for him, both physically and psychologically.

Alex made the baseball team that March. Always an aggressive player, he still knew he had to be careful because his central line was still in his chest. As a first baseman, he had learned early about the importance of diving for balls. As a first baseman with extra "plumbing," he learned how to protect his central line while diving for balls.

Reaching All of His Goals

Alex went to the prom with his best friend, Tracy, and another important goal had been achieved. Each month's visit to the oncologist left Alex and his family holding their breath, fearful of a relapse. Each day was a step closer to graduation.

Graduation day was beautiful. The weather was great, and Alex looked the picture of health—happy and bright-eyed. His oncologist came to the ceremony. They'd become close friends. And when Alex's name was called to receive his diploma, his entire senior class gave him a standing ovation.

While Alex's senior class had been supportive of him, Ellen added, Alex had been an inspiration to them. The most important goals he had set for himself had been met. Now it was time to set more. Alex planned to take a full curriculum at a local community college and then transfer to a university after his first year.

As you can tell from reading about Alex's positive mental attitude, setting goals and working toward them is one way to confront the uncertainties that a cancer diagnosis brings. Listening to the patient's plans for the future and supporting him or her in an optimistic manner go a long way toward making the day-to-day setbacks and discomfort easier to bear for everyone.

How Matt's Family Coped

At two years of age, Matt was too young to set goals or to express how he felt. After his brain tumor surgery and subsequent chemotherapy treatment, Matt couldn't talk at all. But his parents, Sheri and Greg, confronted Matt's cancer head-on.

According to Sheri, she cried a lot, especially the first eighteen months. She cried after treatment was over. And she still cries now. Every three to five months, she "crashes," and then she's okay again.

Matt's older brother, Joey, once asked Sheri why she cries when people mention Matt's name and why she often gets frustrated with Joey at home.

Sheri says that when she thinks back now, she wonders how she would have done on some kind of mood enhancer, something to take the edge off her fears. Sheri says that while she thought about it, she decided against using drugs for several reasons.

Some of the methods Sheri developed for coping were crying, eating, and befriending Matt's medical team. These are common emotional responses to the trauma of caring for a family member being treated for cancer.

Sheri also talked at great length with Matt's nurses, both in the hospital and through home health. Sheri added, "I clearly remember one of our earlier nights at home, and all the trouble Matt was having. The nurse put her arms around me and said, 'this is too much stress for one family to have—take it moment by moment.' I'll never forget that. It was one of the best pieces of advice anyone ever gave me."

The oncology nurses were wonderfully supportive, Sheri recalled. They were patient, understanding, and compassionate. "They knew how to read me and my feelings," Sheri added. "They told me it was okay if I didn't want to or couldn't handle helping with Matt. They only gave me medical and treatment information as I could take it. I came to rely heavily on them for support."

Sometimes, Sheri explained, she actually looked forward to Matt's inpatient treatment sessions so she could be re-energized by certain nurses or doctors. Sheri said that she often sat up very late at night to chat with the night nurse. She lost a lot of sleep, she said, but found this to be very much what she needed at the time.

When well-meaning people suggested that Sheri and Greg "get out" or "take a walk," Sheri said that she couldn't. "I feared for Matt's life if Greg or I was not there with him when something went wrong. It was nerve-wracking to be with him and nerve-wracking not to be. I also felt that Matt had no idea what had happened to him, so how could we 'abandon' him, if only for an hour or two?"

"My husband and I believed that 'this too shall pass,'" Sheri added, "so we survived by thinking we would do everything in our power to get Matt through this crisis." And the family has adjusted its concept of what "happy" means—no cancer. But it's still hard to keep an even emotional keel after nearly four years, Sheri said.

"Now our problems are different ones—rehabilitation and learning issues," Sheri concluded. "Will we ever be situated and happy again? We still long for the 'good old days,' but as Greg frequently points out, we got off the perfect path a long time ago."

When Depression Occurs

The stress of dealing with an illness such as cancer can cause huge emotional upheavals. It can also demand much, both physically and mentally, of everyone whose lives are touched by the cancer diagnosis.

Sometimes, you can get "the blues" for a short period of time. But when these feelings last a long time and interfere with your quality of life, you or someone else in your family may become depressed. When a person is sad, discouraged, pessimistic, despondent, or in despair for several weeks or months, and has trouble managing daily routines, it is possible that he or she is suffering from depression. The bad news is that depression can last a long time if the person doesn't seek help.

In addition to feelings of sadness, symptoms of depression might include trouble with appetite and sleeping, lack of energy, and an inability to concentrate. Alcohol or drug abuse can also be a sign of depression. In extreme cases, depression can lead to thoughts of suicide as a way to end such strong feelings of despair.

Often, a cancer patient focuses all of his or her attention on the cancer. As a result, cancer patients sometimes withdraw from the things they normally enjoy in life—work, social circles and pastimes. The quality of their lives suffers greatly and that encourages their depression.

Depression works like a downward spiral. You feel down, so you don't put any energy into solving problems or facing the stress of coping. Then, when the problems get worse, you feel worse right along with them. This cycling down into depression must be interrupted in some way. Changes have to be made, or you will have these depressed feelings for a long time.

Cancer and Depression

In the cancer patient, depression can be a side effect of some medications, or it can be caused by chemical imbalances that develop because of the cancer.

When cancerous cells invade vital glands such as the pancreas, thyroid, and liver, they can disrupt the normal production of fluids that are needed by the body. Loss of these fluids, such as insulin from the pancreas, in turn causes an imbalance in the chemical makeup of the patient's body. Depending on which glands are affected, and how they interact with each other as well as with the rest of the body, it can cause depression, diabetes, and other problems.

When this happens, adjusting or altering the treatment program may help ease the depression. The oncologist and endocrinologist (blood specialist) work together with the patient to adjust or discontinue any medications that they believe may be contributing to the depression. This is one reason why it's so important for patients to remain in close contact with all the doctors involved in treating their cancer, and to report honestly how they feel.

Some depression is a normal response to the uncertainties of the cancer. It is unrealistic to expect to get rid of all of those feelings. But you can help the patient limit the length and severity of the depression by encouraging your family to work together as a team to deal with the problem.

Enjoyable experiences help cancer patients cope. Having fun makes them feel better, physically and emotionally. When cancer patients are encouraged to do the things they enjoy, it helps them maintain an optimistic attitude. By continuing to do the things they love and to be with people they like, the patient is much less likely to become depressed during really difficult times.

Here are some things you can do to help prevent or alleviate depression while your family copes with cancer.

A. Encourage your sibling or parent to continue doing the things he or she likes best. Playing cards or games, visiting family, doing simple things like going for a drive in the country or a walk in a park with the family can help take the patient's mind off his or her illness. Remind the patient's friends to call or visit often so they can talk about sports, cooking, favorite magazines or books, shopping, and what's happening at school or work. The goal is to keep the patient connected to the rest of the world and participating in those activities that prevent him or her from feeling isolated. It's easy to get depressed when you feel shut out or alone in the world.

B. Do familiar or new things together. You can start a new hobby or collection, put together jigsaw puzzles, or help rearrange the patient's bedroom. You might encourage the patient to keep a journal so he or she can put into words the way he or she feels, or to write poetry. Maybe you like baking cookies together, or searching through old magazines for cool photos. Find new and exciting patterns for needlework by checking out books from your local library. Start a collection of your favorite comic books. Because you know your family member well, you can probably think of many other ways to share time in a creative, positive manner.

C. Even if the patient isn't interested in making things or starting new hobbies, there are still many ways to share quality time together. Watch favorite television shows or rent a funny movie. Listen to good music—the kinds both of you like. Check out joke books from the public library and take turns reading the jokes to each other. Prepare a special dessert that the patient feels like eating, then eat it together in a partylike atmosphere. And don't forget to hold hands and hug each other a lot. A warm, caring touch does a lot to push back the fears and pain of feeling sick.

D. Being hospitalized can cause the patient to become even more depressed. Being away from home—where he or she feels the most secure—can aggravate an already difficult situation. Be the "fun" family member when you visit, the one who arrives with bubbles, silly string, or rub-on tattoos. Life is scary enough for the patient right now without seeing another long face. Take a big sheet of posterboard, painter's tape, and a box of markers or crayons to the hospital. Hang the board so everyone who visits can sign it and leave encouraging messages or draw funny pictures.

Distraction is the name of the game. Having something fun, different, and absorbing to do keeps the patient from dwelling on being sick, frightened, or in pain. Enlist the help of other family members and friends to keep the atmosphere around your home and in the patient's hospital room upbeat and optimistic. Make it a team effort, so you don't feel that all the responsibility for helping the patient avoid depression is on your shoulders.

You should also be aware that living with a person who is depressed can be especially hard on you. It might even lead to your becoming depressed as well. It is important to pay attention to your own emotions as well as helping others in the family. You need to continue doing the things you enjoy in order to maintain a healthy balance in life.

Remember what Sheri said about being afraid to spend time away from Matt? It's a very common feeling. Never forget that you're not alone in this family crisis.

Coping with Hospital Stays and Other Treatment Aspects

It is tough coping with all the changes at home when a family member is diagnosed with cancer. When the person is being treated as an outpatient, you often have more access to the patient, so you will worry less about how he or she is doing. But when that patient must spend days or weeks in the hospital, it may feel scary.

Seeing someone you love surrounded by unfamiliar medical equipment and dozens of strangers, being subjected to harsh chemotherapy treatments and exhaustive physical therapy, may leave you feeling as if all control over your life and your loved one has been lost. Worse, when your family member must travel out of town for highly specialized surgery or treatment, you may feel that kind of anxiety more acutely.

Alex's Hospitalization

"Alex was never hospitalized for just one day. It was always more," his mother, Ellen, said. *"His brothers got used to his being at the hospital, but took comfort in the fact that it was only twenty minutes away from home."*

"Alex had his own way of coping with being hospitalized," Ellen said.

"Alex didn't invite his three brothers to visit, and they didn't go on their own because of it," Ellen added. "Instead, Alex reached inside himself. I was there all the time before work and after working a few hours, in the middle of the night, and often overnight. That's what Alex seemed to need."

When Alex's need for a bone marrow transplant made a trip to Minneapolis a necessity, it was Ellen who went with him. The rest of the family stayed behind. Alex kept in touch with his brothers and school friends by e-mail and telephone calls.

In your family, you may have to feel your way toward complying with what your sick family member wants and needs. Every family copes differently. Ideally, each member of the family finds the role that serves the patient, the family, and himself or herself equally well. But it could take some time. Meanwhile, it helps to know more about what happens in the hospital, what's expected of you, and how to cope when your family member is far away.

Hospital Staff Members and Volunteers Can Make a Huge Difference

While services and amenities may vary from hospital to hospital, the way in which staffers and even the surrounding community respond to the needs of cancer patients and their families is similar in its level of caring and support.

Jan Hagenlocher, public relations director for the Swedish American Hospital in Rockford, Illinois, tells about one case in particular when her coworkers went out of their way.

"A great example is something that occurred last fall. A little girl was dying of cancer here," Jan said. "The staff knew how much she loved animals. Within a few days, we put together her own 'fall festival' and 'petting zoo.' I put the word out, and we ended up with dogs, kittens, bunnies, horses that she got to ride around the parking lot, and even a baby goat."

People responded by donating food and gifts, Jan added. The little girl hadn't smiled in several days, but she did that day. Then, only a few days later, she died.

"This was not just the pediatric staff who got involved, but staff from all across the health system. I know they look at each individual case and do what has to be done," Jan said. "I have observed, on both the adult and pediatric oncology units, that the staff will do whatever it takes to make the patients and their families feel as at-home as can be."

The Swedish American Hospital, as an example, has instituted policies specifically designed to help families cope with long-term hospital stays, Jan explained. In addition to free television and video players, the staff includes round-the-clock pastoral care services and provisions for hairdressing appointments. It also offers discounts on meals, which makes being close to the cancer patient just that much easier.

"Nursing assigns the same caregivers to each patient deliberately, to enhance the feeling of familiarity and continuity of care," Jan added. "Patients are allowed visits from their pets in addition to family members.

"Hospital policies are aimed as much toward improving the patient's mental well-being as their physical health. Volunteers from throughout the community surrounding the hospital provide vital services as well. At Swedish American, volunteers bring mail and floral deliveries to the patient's room, as well as daily newspapers and coffee service.

"We have a strong Candlelighters support group which becomes very involved with families, offering meals, baby-sitting, transportation, and other support. Our child life workers arrange for parties, visits from special people and other social gatherings, and even take patients out on a pass to a movie if it's feasible.

Jan passed on what the Swedish American Hospital's oncology nurses in the pediatric unit felt about supporting patients' families. "In pediatrics, we become very family-oriented with patients who are hospitalized for long periods of time, and with their families," Jan said. "We form close personal relationships. We practice primary care nursing, which then allows the same caregivers to care for the patient, thus building strong continuity in that care."

The pediatric unit has a core group of nurses specifically trained and educated in pediatric oncology. The same is true with the adult oncology units of any hospital. At the Swedish American Hospital, a team that combines pediatric oncology nurses, pediatric social workers, dieticians, child life workers, the hospital chaplain, and a pediatric psychologist meets weekly with the doctors to discuss each patient.

While having a family member staying for long periods at a hospital may at first feel strange, even alien, you'll soon find it can be an open, caring mini-community ready to help you with whatever you and your family need to see this part of cancer treatment through.

Helping Hands for Families Far from Home

When Alex and Ellen traveled to Minneapolis for a bone marrow transplant, they received help from an organization whose name you'll recognize—Ronald McDonald House. It was where the family celebrated Christmas after Alex was released from the hospital but was not ready to go home. Ronald McDonald House provided them with a homelike atmosphere that made Alex's recovery more comfortable.

Back in 1974, when another family was facing the same situation, there were no Ronald McDonald Houses. Fred and Fran Hill spent countless hours over a three-year period, sleeping in a Philadelphia hospital waiting room and eating from vending machines while their daughter, Kim, was undergoing treatment for leukemia.

Fred Hill played for the Philadelphia Eagles football team at the time. With the support of his teammates, Eagles General Manager Jim Murray, and Dr. Audrey Evans from the Children's Hospital of Philadelphia, Fred approached local McDonald's franchises. Together they created Ronald McDonald House. As of 1999, there were 203 of these volunteer-run houses in nineteen countries—all homes away from home that help ease the anxiety of being in a strange city far away from family and friends.

Another group of volunteers offers free air transportation, generally called angel flights, to seriously ill people. As you can imagine, the cost of airplane tickets to fly a patient and family members across the country for treatment can be daunting. That's why several organizations and corporations provide free flights to those in need.

One of these organizations, Dreamline, gives free airline travel for children with serious illnesses, not just for treatment but for fun as well. Another, called the Corporate Angel Network, flies cancer patients and their families to treatment destinations free of charge.

Mercy Medical Airlift is another nonprofit organization dedicated to helping those in compelling need by providing charitable air transportation. Mercy is totally supported through donations plus the services of volunteer pilots and assistants.

And there's one that actually has the name Angel Flights. Like Mercy, Angel Flights is a nonprofit organization of pilots and other volunteers who are dedicated to arranging free private air transportation to patients who cannot afford to use normal commercial airline services. Angel Flights also provides vital help to blood, organ, and tissue banks.

Individual hospitals go out of their way to ease the strain of long-term treatments away from your community. Jan Hagenlocher talked about the Swedish American Hospital's policy toward the families of out-of-town patients.

"Families coming from far away may stay in our hospital hotel rooms, just one floor from the oncology unit," she explained. "We also have hotels nearby that offer low rates and usually free-night stays during the holidays. At Swedish American, we also offer free valet parking and twenty-four-hour visiting except for the pediatrics intensive care unit. But even there, parents may stay overnight in rooms close by."

The hospital helps in other ways, Jan continued. Swedish American provides special parking facilities to accommodate RV hookups. It provides a list of 800-numbers where family members far away can access daily status reports from the nursing staff. And, Jan stressed, oncology case workers, social services, discharge planning, and guest relations staff are always available to help the families in any way they can.

Getting Through the Holidays

The changes that naturally take place in a family coping with cancer seem to become more pronounced during the holidays. While the new experience of having a seriously ill sibling or parent may have become familiar when holiday season rolls around, those special times can loom as a real worry.

As much as you might want to skip any holiday seasons, it's just not possible. The important thing to remember is that you and your family do have options about how to cope. The best thing you can do is to face birthdays, holidays, and other celebrations squarely and plan for what you do or don't want to do to get through these times.

Beloved traditions may have to be set aside because of the patient's illness. Your holiday may be quite different from those you've experienced in the past. You may have to miss family gatherings that require travel. Your family may have to cut back on decorating, baking, or celebrating at the level you'd normally expect at home. But that doesn't mean the holidays have to be less meaningful or fun.

And, you might be surprised. If the patient is home and doing well, changes may be minimal. What's important is that you and your family talk honestly and openly about what each member wants and needs to make the holidays more bearable and meaningful. It may take some compromise and negotiation. Flexibility is the key, as well as remembering that this is a temporary situation. It's just one holiday or birthday out of the many you'll share with your family in the years to come.

You can start the process by talking about the holidays and your expectations. Discuss what you're looking forward to most, what you are not looking forward to, what would make the day special for you, and which traditions you want to see continued. Encourage the other family members to share their concerns and wishes.

Holidays with Alex and His Family

Thanksgiving and Christmas were Alex's favorite holidays, his mother, Ellen, recalled. While next-oldest brother Forrest had more or less outgrown holidays, for Danny and Lucas, Christmas was still their favorite.

"We've never held to a lot of tradition other than a big meal at Thanksgiving, with a lot of choices, based on what the boys thought would be good," Ellen added. "Decorating the tree at Christmas time is our most cherished tradition."

After Alex's original diagnosis, the holidays became even more important to each individual and the family as a unit, Ellen explained.

"We wanted to make it the best because we didn't know what the next year would bring," she said. "The first holiday season, Alex targeted those two holidays as the ones he most wanted to be home for, and he succeeded."

That Thanksgiving, the family enjoyed a traditional turkey dinner, with their favorite cookies and pies.

"For Christmas, we had homemade pizza," Ellen remembered. "We all savored the slower pace of the day. Alex had just been discharged a couple of days before and was still on a lot of medication."

Instead of a natural Christmas tree, the family decorated an artificial one. Alex was too vulnerable to infections to have a real tree brought into his home environment. Ellen said that even their house plants were being baby-sat in other homes in order to protect Alex.

But when Alex and Ellen spent the next Christmas season in Minneapolis after he underwent the bone marrow transplant, Ellen said, the spirit of the holiday went with them.

"We all celebrated in Minneapolis, but Alex's father and brothers did nothing as far as decorating at home," Ellen added. "It didn't feel right to them."

Asked if the family made any changes, Ellen said, "If you had known Alex, you would have seen how important it was for him that things be as normal as they could be. It kept him focused. His cancer was always 'under foot,' but he was determined it wouldn't be in charge of his life."

In respect of Alex's wishes, Ellen explained that the rest of the family tried to keep things as normal as they could. For example, in his role as eldest child, Alex passed out the Christmas gifts one at a time, just as he'd done for years.

"The one thing Alex's brothers did differently was to let Alex know in every way possible how much they loved him, wanted to help him, and wanted to

care for him," Ellen said. "When we were in Minneapolis, they let Alex know how much they missed him. For all their usual sibling bickering, they were now behaving as a solid unit."

Holidays with Matt and His Family

When Matt was first diagnosed and was in treatment for eighteen months, holidays came and went, Sheri said. The family's only goal was to get through each and every day, counting down to the end of treatment.

"We fully expected to be in the hospital on any given holiday," Sheri added. "If we weren't, we stayed put at home so we were just a phone call away from the doctor and a short distance from the hospital if we needed to take Matt in."

Matt was too fragile and too loaded with equipment to go anywhere but the hospital for the first year, Sheri explained. Matt's home was too small to entertain the entire family at holidays. With the dining room taken over as a hospital room, there was even less space to accommodate guests.

"That first Christmas while Matt was in treatment, our families made visits to our house throughout Christmas week," Sheri said. "We had always been accustomed to going to other family members' homes for holiday celebrations. The only change was that we stayed home and they came to visit us in small doses, so to speak."

Matt's aunt lived close by and hosted many holidays in a row to make it easier, Sheri added. Other family members traveled from outside the immediate area to spend the holidays near Matt. Sheri's sisters did the Easter shopping for the family.

"The kids loved the baskets, and they even remembered Greg and me," Sheri recalled. "I got a new tube of lipstick and a pair of earrings. It was so thoughtful of them."

It felt safe to be just with immediate family the first two years, Sheri remembered. But now that Matt is recovering, holidays can still be hard.

"This past Christmas was particularly difficult when we were with family," Sheri said. "Matt is doing so well in so many areas that I tend to forget how far behind he really is in his development and abilities."

Sheri's extended family includes eleven grandchildren under the age of nine, with most of them boys between the ages of five and nine, she explained. While the other boys, so close in age and interests, were running here, there, up and down, Matt sat on the family room floor looking at picture books and playing with toys designed for kids much younger than he is.

"We'd put in a movie for him. Someone would come and switch the television over to a football game," Sheri said. "No one seemed to notice how isolated Matt was. If Greg or I wasn't on the floor, interacting with him, he was on his own."

It wasn't intentional, of course, but it was hurtful to Matt, Sheri added. Because Matt still needed so much help getting around and up stairs, by the time his parents took him to where the action was, the other boys had moved on to something else, somewhere else in the house.

"I cried on and off that whole day," Sheri recalled. *"I would slip into the bathroom to wipe my eyes, blow my nose, take a deep breath, and go back at it."*

Despite understanding that Matt will never be the same, Sheri said holidays have become more cheerful now that Matt is beginning to improve.

"They're different but they're still fun," Sheri added. *"Thinking about Halloween costumes in August is really very normal. The kids plan and plan what they're going to be. It's uplifting to finally have Matt so tuned in to what everyone else is talking about, and doing what they're doing."*

The family has adjusted holiday plans to fit Matt's abilities, Sheri said.

"Matt's birthday parties revolve around things that are more sedentary for everyone, such as bowling, parties at home, or popular, kid-oriented restaurants such as Chuck E. Cheese. We try to do things where there is forced socialization. That way, Matt isn't just surrounded by adults. It's become a natural way of planning."

What You Can Do to Cope with Holiday Celebrations

It may sound strange, but younger people are often able to separate their anxiety about a family member's illness from the joy of the season. This doesn't mean they don't care. On the other hand, you and the adult members of your family will more keenly feel the intrusion of cancer on the holiday atmosphere.

When the patient is home during holidays and birthdays, being together and celebrating can be especially satisfying in spite of the compromises and changes that might need to be made. But if the patient is hospitalized when the celebrations roll around, as in Alex's case that second Christmas, it is probably going to be tough. Facing this situation squarely and dealing with it is your best option.

If the hospital is near your home, you and your family can plan many activities and visits to make the holidays enjoyable, even if it differs from your traditional celebration.

Hospitals go out of their way to make holidays and birthdays bright and cheery for patients who can't go home to celebrate. Jan Hagenlocher from the Swedish American Hospital said all of the holidays are celebrated in a meaningful, appropriate manner.

"At Christmas, we have Santa and carolers. We have a large party, partially sponsored by the Make-A-Wish Foundation," Jan explained. "The hospital has many, many local people who want to donate money, gifts, treats, and more. The hallways are all brightly decorated."

In addition to a large bulletin board that changes decorations with the passing holidays, Jan said the Swedish American sponsors an Easter egg hunt with a visit from the Easter Bunny. The hospital staff plans picnics during the summer months. And on Halloween, the young patients "trick or treat" to the various departments in the hospital.

Special menus in the hospital's restaurant invite everyone at the hospital to enter into the spirit of the holiday, she added. Patients and their families are allowed to add to each room's decorations as long as they comply with any infection-control issues.

"Our Candlelighters group provides a lot of the support for these celebrations," Jan said. "The entire hospital staff is especially sensitive to patients during holiday seasons. We also attempt to address unique cultural and spiritual needs as well, if the family asks."

There are a number of things you can do to bring the joys of any holiday with you to the hospital. Most provide VCR equipment and television sets in each room. You can bring or rent the patient's favorite holiday videos to share. If the patient is your brother or sister, ask his or her friends to do the same. Spending quiet time enjoying a favorite holiday movie or television special is a comforting way to share the fun.

Holiday or birthday cards are another way to brighten up those special days. You can bring the family's Christmas cards in to share. Ask the hospital staff how best to hang or display cards in the patient's room. If the patient is a sibling, talk to his or her teacher about having classmates make special cards. Or you can bring construction paper, crayons, and other supplies to the hospital so your family member can make cards to send to friends and other family members.

Help your hospitalized family member "go shopping" for little holiday gifts by bringing in advertising flyers from the local newspaper. Once the surprises are chosen, ask the parent of a friend to take you shopping. After you have completed the shopping, you and the patient can spend a long winter afternoon having a "wrap party."

If the patient is a younger sibling or relative, find a new coloring book that focuses on the holiday and bring it along when you visit. Or borrow a new holiday storybook from the library to read together.

Even the simplest activities can help alleviate the strangeness of spending a holiday or birthday at the hospital. Discovering new activities and sharing the fun will help lift everyone's spirits. The important thing is not to let a change in the way your family celebrates a holiday keep you from making the most of it.

Coping with Cancer's Long-Term Effects

Fairy tales begin with "once upon a time" and usually end with everyone living happily ever after. When you are coping with cancer in your family, you need to understand that it is highly unlikely that there will be a perfectly happy ending.

At the very best, your sibling or parent will survive cancer and its treatments, and go on to live a full, productive life. However, it is also quite likely that your family member will survive cancer with some impairment, and live the rest of his or her life with the possibility of the cancer reoccurring. At the very worst, you'll lose your loved one.

Researchers have made amazing strides in diagnosing and treating cancer, dramatically improving the patient's odds of survival. Through genetic engineering, scientists are even narrowing down the possibility of preventing cancers from ever starting. Still, cancer takes its daily toll. There's a lot more research to be done before the long-term results of a cancer diagnosis are more positive than negative.

Coping with Loss: The End of Alex's Story

Alex seemed to be recovering well from his bone marrow transplant, which took place in December

1998. But in March, his mother, Ellen, noticed some changes that really worried her.

"Alex's grandfather died from colon cancer in February. The mothers of two of Alex's friends arrived to take care of him while I went to the funeral," Ellen said. "I was gone for a week. Within a few days of my return, I noticed Alex was sleeping more than usual."

Ellen recalled that she was determined to keep him awake, fearing that Alex was suffering from lack of motivation, boredom, and possibly depression.

"There was something wrong with the way Alex was sleeping all the time," Ellen added. "He didn't wake up to eat. Getting medications into him was a major task. We went for a drive that Sunday, and I had to practically drag him out of his room. Alex got snappish, then really quiet. After an hour's drive, we came home. Alex's mood was no better, and that just wasn't like him at all."

Upon hearing these symptoms, Alex's doctor told Ellen to bring him into the clinic early the next day for an MRI. By that time, Alex's speech was like that of a movie slowed down to quarter-speed, Ellen remembered. Alex was hospitalized again. He became unresponsive and lost control of his bodily functions. A few days later, Alex was diagnosed with Epstein-Barr encephalitis, a serious viral infection.

"It took Alex three weeks to remember who I was, and another seven weeks before he was strong enough to leave the hospital," Ellen said.

During the months following his release, Alex's condition slowly began to deteriorate again. By September, Alex needed round-the-clock care. At one time or another, Ellen said, his brothers each asked about the possibility of Alex's dying.

"Although at the times they asked, his condition didn't make that seem an imminent possibility," Ellen explained. "I cautioned them all that something could come up that we weren't expecting."

All three brothers visited a neuropsychologist before Alex's death, Ellen added.

"I said good-bye to Alex every day starting in March when he was hospitalized for encephalitis, never knowing if he would come out of it," Ellen recalled. "When he started failing again in July, I knew the downward spiral would continue. My good-byes centered on telling Alex much I loved him, giving him hugs, and respecting him. Telling him again and again how proud I was of him, and how he had never disappointed me."

Ellen said she did everything she could to comfort Alex and ease his pain, including tolerating his mood swings.

"I accepted Alex's tiredness for what it was, the end of a long, hard road," Ellen remembered.

Alex died on December 7, 1999.

The dynamics in Alex's family have changed with his passing, Ellen observed.

"While Danny and Lucas know that Forrest has always been an older brother, I think part of the rivalry is because now he's the only older brother," Ellen said. "There was a lot of respect for Alex even when they weren't getting along, so he left a big set of shoes to fill. Forrest tried to fill those shoes as a child when he followed Alex around.

He experienced a lot of heartache until he learned he was his own person."

Forrest also had major problems with migraines up until Alex's death. Ellen said that after Alex died, Forrest's migraines subsided in numbers and strength, and he was able to start attending school more regularly.

"One of the hardest things he has recently dealt with is becoming the oldest brother," Ellen said. "It's a job/title/position Forrest never wanted, and one he doesn't feel right holding."

Another difficult situation Alex's brothers had to face was lack of understanding from their schools, Ellen explained.

"We need to remind communities, teachers, and counselors specifically, that recovery from a death takes time," Ellen said. "Whether we expect it or not, whether it is a parent or sibling, we need time. I'd ask that you put yourself in the other person's shoes before judging."

Ellen said she had experienced some problems with a few of the boys' teachers who seemed to expect more of their students than they would of themselves or of their peers.

"Some of the boys' teachers seem to expect them to 'bounce back' right away. Just a little understanding and acknowledgment that there will be rough days would help," Ellen added. "There's a lot of grief in trying to recover from a hugely traumatic loss."

When someone asks her how many children she has, Ellen said in her heart the answer will always be four.

"In reality there are only three now," Ellen said. "That comes back to the boys, too. A nurse friend suggested responding four, and providing further details. It's good advice that I know I'll use. I feel strongly that ignoring or eliminating Alex from the family makes his loss all the harder to accept."

The knowledge that Alex has been an inspiration to so many helps, Ellen added.

"I heard through Forrest that a young man going out to play first base for the varsity baseball team was told by the coach to watch videos of Alex playing," Ellen explained. "Alex would have been thrilled to hear that."

Ellen also feels strongly about what she believes is a lack of research and support for young cancer victims. This feeling has grown not only out of her loss but from what she discovered during personal research and experiences while Alex was being treated.

"We hear a lot about AIDS. We hear the president talking about increasing AIDS funding," Ellen said. "There isn't a single soul in Washington talking about increasing funding for childhood cancer research and cures. We're not hearing a thing about the fourteen- to nineteen-year-old age bracket getting cancer with less chances of survival than the other age brackets for children. Why?"

Ellen added she was shocked and appalled to learn that pediatric AIDS research is funded at four times the level of pediatric cancer research.

"Don't misunderstand—treating all childhood diseases is important, but can't we even the playing field a little?" Ellen asked. "Danny Thomas and St. Jude's

did a lot for raising awareness and fund-raising, but what about a national agenda?"

To understand more clearly, Ellen suggested going to any hospital with a pediatric oncology unit and seeing firsthand the "hell" those children go through.

"Really see these children, from those who haven't yet learned to talk so they can't ask why, to those who know only too well what the odds are and are afraid to ask all the questions," Ellen said.

Even if you're not moved by the loss of a family member to examine cancer funding and medical advances more closely, there are things you can do at home to help get through these difficult times.

One method suggested by the Pediatric Oncology Resource Center for getting through especially tough times is called the Three Ts.

A. Touching: Tender touching says "I love you and I care." Everyone in your family needs to be touched and held. Younger siblings especially need to be hugged, held, and cuddled. Strong arms feel secure when your world is falling apart. A three-minute hug is a good idea.

B. Tears: Everyone needs to be able to cry and know it's okay. Everyone in the family needs to know that they don't have to be afraid of tears.

C. Talking: All of your family will need to talk. Listen with your heart to your parents and siblings. Younger siblings especially need to know they were not to blame, that other family members are unlikely to die, and that there will always be someone to love and care for them.

Matt's Recovery: Celebrating Small Miracles

"Matt walks! Matt walks!" That was the e-mail Sheri and Greg sent to family, friends, and Candlelighters members in January 2000. For the first time in the nearly four years since he was diagnosed with a brain tumor at age two, Matt was able to take a few precious steps unassisted.

"I'm so proud of him," Sheri said. "Never in a million years would I have thought that these little things would be such big things, nor would I have ever thought that they'd take so long to achieve.

"Matt will go to school tomorrow on a suburban instead of a wheelchair bus. He will be able to walk down the hotel hallway this weekend holding his nine-year-old cousin's hand instead of an adult's. These are the tiny, remarkable things we no longer take for granted. These are Matt's milestones."

It was just a short time before, at Christmas, that Sheri agonized over Matt's isolation and limitations as she compared him to his cousins.

"It was just so striking to me that Matt would never be able to keep up with his peers and, unless it was facilitated by an adult, he would not have playmates who sought him out," Sheri remembered.

His cancer had taken away his mobility for years. Sheri is still concerned that the brain damage Matt received from the cancer and surgery may prevent him from being actively social with his peer group in unstructured settings.

"His speech is still somewhat difficult to understand to the untrained ear, and his volume is not readily heard," Sheri added. "Kids often don't even realize he is attempting to get in on the conversation or activity."

Sheri explained that she and Greg had expected full recovery from the brain tumor for Matt, but it still looks as if they won't get it.

"Our baseline for Matt has changed radically from what we originally knew of him before his tumor," Sheri added. "Because it has become so normal to us, it was quite devastating to me to see just how impaired he really is when I saw him beside my nephews who are his age."

Recent breakthroughs in medical treatment have changed the focus for families who are coping with cancer. Instead of dealing with a life-threatening illness, now they are learning how to cope after the treatment is completed, as in Matt's case.

All the fears, stress, and changes that take place during active cancer therapy are to be expected. Those that accompany long-term recovery aren't so obvious, but they are just as real. You'll have many questions about your family member's cure and long-term survival. It may be a rough transition.

At first, you may feel as if your whole life has been disrupted again, just as it was when your parent or sibling was diagnosed. You've already dealt with the shock and fears, treatment schedules, hospitalization, and clinic visits. You've accepted the changes that have had to be made at home. And you've established relationships with the medical staff who treated your family member. All those things that disrupted your life have become routine and ordinary.

Now that treatment is complete, it's all going to change again, but it will never change back to the way things were before cancer invaded your home. Instead, you are facing a new order, one you might not be prepared to accept. And it's going to be hard to explain that to other family members.

Some of those initial fears may persist. You might worry about the patient relapsing without the protection of treatment. Talking to an oncology social worker or to the hospital staff who treated the patient will help soothe those fears. After all, the patient's ongoing condition will be closely monitored for months and even years to come. There will be regular follow-up testing, and physical therapy may also continue for a long time.

You've read in previous chapters that providing as normal an atmosphere as possible for the patient during treatment is vital. It's just as important after the treatments end and the patient is on the mend. The relationship you share with the patient should continue as it was, but the focus should begin to change.

The patient should attend regular family functions such as holiday gatherings, picnics, religious services, and reunions. A return to school and assigned chores is another signal that the patient is ready to resume a normal lifestyle. Reasonable and fair amounts of attention are part of the transition, as is encouraging the patient to live up to normal expectations.

If the patient is a child or teen, don't be surprised if he or she goes through a period of withdrawal from all the attention received while being treated. The patient may need time to adjust physically and emotionally to not being the center of attention, plus having to deal with the real world again.

Don't be surprised if other family members, friends, and neighbors don't call or drop by as often. They may feel that, with the immediate crisis past, their constant presence is no longer needed. If you feel you still need their support, keep in touch through phone calls and get-togethers. Don't stop attending the support groups that helped you through the hardest days. You may still need them even though the worst is over.

Most important, all of your family members need to be encouraged to talk about their concerns. The goal is to bring the patient, as well as his or her family members, back into the mainstream of life.

Because they are the mothers of children with cancer, Ellen and Sheri felt the effects intensely. The way in which they have chosen to deal with these "leftover" emotions is to become involved as volunteers. You've just read how Ellen feels about the lack of research and funding available for childhood cancers. Her reaction has been to help by researching and reporting new findings and information to a local cancer support organization.

Sheri's volunteer efforts began in January 1999, when she and other parents of children with cancer were approached by one of the hospital's oncologists to revive the Candlelighters support group.

"Candlelighters had waxed and waned through the years," Sheri explained. "We were all at different stages of our kids' diagnosis but were very honored to be approached. My son had just completed treatment, and two of the parents had lost their children."

With the child life specialist joining them as a hospital liaison, Sheri said, the volunteers went to work identifying what the group could do for each other, finding newly diagnosed families, and those who will always be "burning the candle." Together, they mapped out a year of social events and support meetings.

"It was a very exciting year, to find out what each family needed, as identified by their attendance at the various events and functions," Sheri added. "We have a steady group of six families who always participate. I have been voted president, followed by three other officer positions. I am grateful to have this position, as I have a strong desire to provide outreach support to families, especially new ones."

One year later, the relationship between Candlelighters and its oncology team has grown into a partnership. These dedicated medical professionals refer new families to Candlelighters soon after diagnosis.

"Most of us 'oldtimers' did not have an opportunity to be part of such a group," Sheri commented. "This position also enables me to approach the doctors from an advisee position as well as a parent. Candlelighters has helped me maintain my relationship with them, making me feel comfortable that my son is still important in their eyes even though we're a few years out of treatment."

Through Candlelighters, the relationship Sheri developed with Matt's oncologists continues to give her the emotional support she feels she needs. Being involved with the support group assures her that everyone is still committed to all of the children and their families, regardless of how frequently they may see them.

"My association with the national Candlelighters group has been mainly on-line," Sheri explained. "But their response to requests for material (resources) has been the biggest advantage. We can put books into the hands of some very scared, devastated parents."

The national group gives Sheri's local chapter name recognition, although Sheri noted that childhood cancer groups are little-known outside of their immediate circle. Still, Sheri regularly corresponds by e-mail with other parents of cancer patients worldwide.

"St. Jude's continues to get the media coverage and financial support, even from local businesses," Sheri added. "We would like to increase our visibility and awareness so we may attract that attention to our own group and treatment center."

As you can understand, concerns and thoughts about cancer don't stop when the treatments end, nor when the patient is pronounced "cured." As one pessimistic person on the Internet put it, "I've been told the only way a person will be considered cured of cancer is if he or she dies from some other cause."

More and more, that is not the case. But the main thing to remember is that you have options and choices in how you cope with cancer in your family. How you decide to deal with this challenge now that you know more about it is very much up to you.

Glossary

anesthesia Loss of sensation or consciousness induced by specialized drugs or, in some cases, by disease.

biopsy Removal of samples of living tissue and fluids for diagnostic examinations.

chemotherapy Prevention or treatment of disease through the systematic administering of chemicals.

hematology Branch of medicine that deals with diseases of the blood, such as leukemia.

Hodgkin's disease Disease in which lymph nodes throughout the body become progressively enlarged and inflamed.

interferon Cellular protein induced in response to infection by a virus that acts to slow the virus's growth.

interleukin Compound produced by lymphocytes and other cells that helps regulate immune responses.

leukemia Any one of a group of diseases that attack the organs that produce blood, often accompanied by anemia and the enlargement of the lymph nodes, spleen, and liver.

lumbar Term designating the vertebrae, nerves, arteries, and other vital organs in the lower portion of the body's trunk.

lymphocytic Describes a variety of blood-based cells formed in lymphatic tissue, important in the creation of antibodies.

malignant Anything dangerous or virulent, which causes or is likely to cause death.

necrosis The death or decay of tissue in a particular part of the body.

neurologist Specialist in the branch of medicine dealing with the nervous system, including its structure and diseases.

neutrophil Type of white blood cell in spinal blood that can easily be stained by neutral dyes.

oncology The branch of medicine dealing with tumors, including cancers.

palliation The relief of pain or the alleviation of the severity of a disease, such as cancer, without actually curing it.

pediatrics The branch of medicine dealing with the development and care of infants and children, and with the treatment of childhood diseases.

prognosis The prediction of the probable course of a disease and the chances of recovery.

pulmonary Refers to the lungs, as well as the system of arteries and veins that carry blood from the heart to the lungs and back.

sepsis Poisoned condition caused by the absorption of toxic microorganisms and their by-products into the bloodstream.

tracheotomy Surgical incision into the throat area to create an artificial breathing hole.

Where to Go for Help

You'll find that there is an amazing, almost overwhelming amount of information on every facet of cancer available at your school and public library, as well as from cancer support organizations and on-line. It will help if you narrow your focus to the particular type of cancer your family member has. As far as understanding treatment processes, coping with changes, and what to expect, the resources available are almost unlimited.

Here, then, is a starter list based on the sources the author used while researching and writing this book. From here, you can go to thousands of sites on-line. Ask your school or public librarian for more suggestions in fiction and nonfiction reading to support your search for information on coping with cancer in your family.

You can also contact the hospitals in your community for information on support groups. The hospitals the author worked with offered between one and six different groups, each centered on an age or type of cancer. All of them were very actively involved in helping families cope with cancer and with all its emotional and spiritual upheavals.

Support Organizations and Resources

Associations in the United States

The American Cancer Society
(800) ACS-2345 (227-2345)
The above telephone number will help you reach the society's
national headquarters in the United States. Look in your telephone book to find the local chapter. Both national and local
sources are very generous in the materials they provide and
helpful in finding more information.
Web site: http://www.cancer.org

American Dietetic Association
216 West Jackson Boulevard
Chicago, IL 60606-6995
(312) 899-0040
Web site: http://www.eatright.org

Candlelighters Childhood Cancer Foundation
Look in the telephone directory for the chapter nearest to you.
This support group was founded in 1970, and now totals
nearly 45,000 members. Alex's and Matt's families are
among them. Candlelighters produces free publications
which are excellent reference materials written for parents
and older children. They also produce a newsletter which
spotlights current practices, legislature, and personal stories
as well as ideas on continued support of families coping
with childhood cancer.

National Cancer Institute
NCI Public Inquiries Office
Building, 31, Room 10A03
31 Center Drive, MSC 2580

Bethesda, MD 20892-2580
(301) 435-3848
Web site: http://www.nci.nih.gov

National Coalition for Cancer Survivorship
1010 Wayne Avenue
Suite 770
Silver Spring, MD 20910-5600
(877) NCCS YES (622-7937)
Web site: http://www.cansearch.org
e-mail: info@cansearch.org

The National Hospice and Palliative Care Organization
(800) 658-8898
This organization of volunteers provides quality compassionate care at the end of life. Either its members come to your home, or the patient is lodged in a home-like setting where both patient and family receive emotional and spiritual support. Look in your telephone directory for a local chapter.

Associations in Canada

Canadian Cancer Society
10 Alcorn Avenue, Suite 200
Toronto, ON M4V 3B1
(416) 961-7223
(888) 939-3333
Web site: http://www.cancer.ca

The Childhood Cancer Foundation—Candlelighters Canada
55 Eglinton Avenue East, Suite 401
Toronto, ON M4P 1GB
(800) 363-1062

National Cancer Institute of Canada
10 Alcorn Avenue, Suite 20
Toronto, ON M4V 3B1
(416) 961-7223
Closely aligned with the Canadian Cancer Society, NCIC
supports cancer research and related programs.

Wellspring Cancer Support Centre
81 Wellesley Street East
Toronto, ON M4Y 1H6
(416) 961-1928
Wellspring offers a range of support programs both onsite
and on-line.

Web Sites in the United States

Association of Cancer Online Resources
http://www.acor.org

Cancer Care, Inc.
http://www.cancercare.org

Cancer Information and Support International
http://www.cancer-info.com

Cancer News on the Net
http://www.cancernews.com

Cancer Resources
http://www.cancerresources.com

The Cancer Support Network
http://www.cancersupportnetwork.org

Cancer Wellness Center
http://www.cancerwellness.org

Candlelighters Childhood Cancer Foundation
http://www.candlelighters.org
http://www.candlelightstories.com
Log on here for firsthand stories about cancer in children, and
their families.

Kids With Cancer
http://www.kidswithcancer.com

The Leukemia and Lymphoma Society
http://www.leukemia.org
Here you'll find specific information on blood-borne cancers
with a multitude of links to specific data sites.

The National Hospice and Palliative Care Organization
http://www.nho.org

The Neverending Squirrel Tale
http://www.squirreltales.com

Pediatric Oncology Resource Center
http://www.acor.org/diseases/ped-onc
e-mail: info@cancercare.org

The University of Pennsylvania Cancer Center
http://www.oncolink.upenn.edu

The Wellness Community
http://www.twcdel.org

Web Sites in Canada

British Columbia Cancer Agency
http://www.bccancer.bc.ca

Canadian Cancer Research Group
http://www.ccrg.com

Cancer Organizations in Canada
http://www.healthcastle.com/org_canada.shtml

CanSurmount
http://www.islandnet.com/CanSurmount
Headquartered in Victoria, British Columbia, CanSurmount is
a network of cancer survivors whose experiences and insights
provide inspiration and assistance to those facing the
same challenges.

The Childhood Cancer Foundation—Candlelighters Canada
http://www.candlelighters.ca
Visit http://www.candlelightstories.com for firsthand stories
about cancer in children and their families.

Families of Children with Cancer (FCC) Canada
http://www.fcco.org
Based in the Toronto Hospital for Sick Children, FCC provides
educational materials, as well as support groups and an advo-
cacy program.

National Cancer Institute of Canada
http://www.ncic.cancer.ca

Wellspring Cancer Support Centre
http://www.wellspring.ca

Angel Flight

Angel Flight is one of a number of nonprofit organizations made up of pilots and other volunteers who arrange free private air transportation for medical patients who cannot afford to use commercial flights. It is a member of Air Care Alliance, (http://www.aircareall.org/) and is coordinated through:

National Patient Air Transport
(800) 296-1217

Other contacts include:
AirLifeline at (800) 446-1231 or (916) 641-7800

Continental Careforce at (713) 438-0376:
contact Bob Jack

Corporate Angels at (914) 328-1313

Lifeline Pilots at (800) 822-7972

Wings of Freedom at (407) 363-1991

For Further Reading

Aker, Saundra, N., and Polly Lenssen. *A Guide to Good Nutrition During and After Chemotherapy and Radiation.* Seattle, WA: Fred Hutchinson Cancer Research Center, 1998.

American Cancer Society. *It Helps to Have Friends. What Happened to You, Happened to Me. Caring for the Patient with Cancer at Home. After Diagnosis: A Guide for Patients and Families. When Your Brother or Sister Has Cancer. Listen with Your Heart.*
Call the national headquarters at (800) ACS-2345 or contact your local American Cancer Society chapter for copies of these informative books and pamphlets.

Capossela, Cappy, and Sheila Warnock. *Share the Care: How to Organize a Group to Care for Someone Who is Seriously Ill.* New York: Simon and Schuster, 1995.

Dollinger, Malin, MD, Ernest H. Rosenbaum, and Greg Cable, eds. *Everyone's Guide to Cancer Therapy.* Kansas City, MO: Andrews & McMeel Publishing, 1998.

Harpham, Wendy Schlessel. *After Cancer : A Guide to Your New Life.* New York: HarperPerennial, 1995

McKay, Judith, and Nancee Hirano. *The Chemotherapy &
Radiation Therapy Survival Guide*. Oakland, CA: New
Harbinger Publications, 1998.

Morra, Marion, and Eve Potts. *Choices*. New York: Avon
Books, 1994.

Nathan, Joel. *What to Do When They Say "It's Cancer."* St.
Leonards, NSW, Australia: Allen and Unwin, 1999.
Australian Joel Nathan was given months to live after his
cancer diagnosis, but he has survived for more than sixteen
years. What he has to say about this experience may give you
insight into the long-term aspect of cancer recovery.

Pennebaker, Ruth. *Both Sides Now*. New York: Henry Holt &
Company, 2000.
A down-to-earth teen's life is turned upside-down when her
mother is diagnosed with breast cancer. This straight-talking
novel looks at the changes cancer brings through both the
mother's and daughter's eyes.

Rando, Therese A., Ph.D. *How to Go on Living When
Someone You Love Dies*. New York: Bantam
Books, 1991.
This is one of many excellent books that deals with the loss of a
loved one to cancer. A bereavement specialist, Rando gently
leads readers through the painful process that follows the loss of
a loved one.

Schimmel, Selma R., with Barry Fox. *CancerTalk: Voices of
Hope and Endurance from "The Group Room," the
World's Largest Cancer Support Group*. New York:
Broadway Books, 1999.

Trillin, Alice. *Dear Bruno.* New York: New Press, 1996.
Author Alice Trillon, an adult cancer patient, wrote this series of letters to a friend's teenage son, who was also battling cancer. The letters deal with issues surrounding living with a cancer diagnosis in a frank, honest, and sometimes humorous manner.

Wolford, Charles B., with Faye Wolford. *My Story About Cancer.* New York: Seven Locks Press, 1999.
This short but very moving book was written by Charles after he was diagnosed with cancer at age fourteen. When he died fifteen months later, his mother finished the last few pages. In this journal, Charles talks candidly about his fears and feelings.

Index